Energy Diagnostic and Treatment Methods

Also by Fred P. Gallo

Energy Psychology: Explorations at the Interface of
Energy, Cognition, Behavior, and Health

A NORTON PROFESSIONAL BOOK

Energy Diagnostic and Treatment Methods

Fred P. Gallo, Ph.D.

W. W. Norton & Company
New York • London

To contact the author for further information about workshops, presentations, seminars, and educational materials, write to Psychological Services, 40 Snyder Road, Hermitage, PA 16148. You may also call (724-346-3838), fax (724-346-4339), or E-mail (fgallo@energypsych.com). Visit the author's Web site: www.energypsych.com.

For information about permission to reproduce selections
from this book, write to
Permissions, W. W. Norton & Company, Inc., 500 Fifth Avenue,
New York, NY 10110

Composition by Bytheway Publishing Services
Manufacturing by Haddon Craftsmen

Library of Congress Cataloging-in-Publication Data

Gallo, Fred P.
   Energy diagnostic and treatment methods / Fred P. Gallo
        p.   cm.
      "A Norton professional book."
      Includes bibliographical references and index.
      ISBN 0-393-70312-6
   1. Bioenergetic psychotherapy.   2. Mind and body therapies.   I. Title.

RC489.B5 G345   2000
616.89'14 — dc21   99-049653

W. W. Norton & Company, Inc., 500 Fifth Avenue, New York, N.Y. 10110
www.wwnorton.com

W. W. Norton & Company Ltd., 10 Coptic Street, London WC1A 1PU

2   3   4   5   6   7   8   9   0

To My Parents

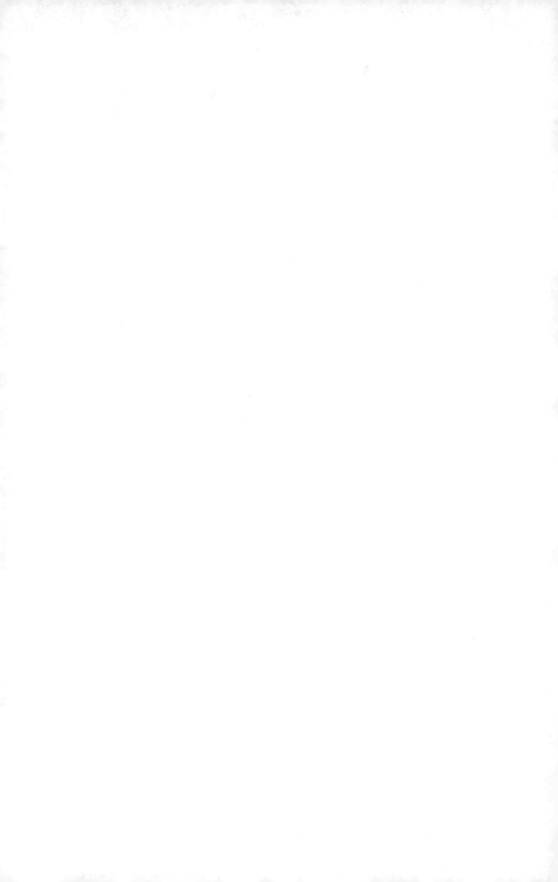

CONTENTS

ACKNOWLEDGMENTS

A BOOK SELDOM STANDS alone. It has a rhizome that penetrates into the soil, through which it obtains nutrients. In this way it grows, aided by the light of a star toward which it aspires. Even that which is offered as something new grows from ground previously seeded and plowed. As Harry S. Truman said, "There is nothing new in the world except the history you do not know." Therefore I acknowledge those directly, indirectly, unknowingly, and unknown who contributed to the creation of this work.

In the known column I would like to recognize the contributions of Huang Ti, George J. Goodheart, Jr., Florence and Harry Kendall, John Thie, Alan Beardall, Gordon Stokes, Daniel Whiteside, David S. Walther, Paul and Gail Dennison, John Diamond, Roger J. Callahan, James V. Durlacher, Francine Shapiro, Robert O. Becker, Harold Saxon Burr, Rupert Sheldrake, David Bohm, Gary Craig, Carl Rogers, Abraham Maslow, Edmund Husserl, Martin Buber, Richard Bandler, John Grinder, Robert Dilts, and Milton H. Erickson.

I would also like to thank Michael Formica for his expertise in the areas of physics and computer science, and his patience with my lack thereof; Amy Formica for her assistance with photographs; and a whole host of others too numerous to mention.

Thank you to all the talented people at W. W. Norton, and special appreciation to Leeann Graham and to Susan Munro for contacting and supporting me throughout this project. Also, I wish to express my gratitude to those who have corresponded with me and attended my seminars. Their comments and questions helped me hone the ideas and methods presented in this book. Thanks to my good friend, John Frisco, for inspiring conversations and mutual exploration that have been abundantly helpful.

INTRODUCTION

Man's mind stretched to a new idea never
goes back to its original dimension.

— *Oliver Wendell Holmes*

IN 1992, I read an article describing a technique that purported to reduce
addictive cravings. The author proposed that cravings are consistent with
anxiety and that his technique treated the underlying cause of the anxiety,
which he claimed to occur within a bodily energy system, at a level more
basic than cognition. While much of this made sense to me in light of
my clinical experience with addictive disorders, particularly the suggested
relationship between addictive cravings and anxiety, I found the treatment
that he offered to be quite unusual to say the least! He recommended
that the addicted person tap directly under an eye, followed by tapping
approximately four inches under an armpit. I remember laughing at the
suggestion after tapping at those locations myself to make sure I had it right.
I then placed the article among a pile of papers on a shelf in my study
and essentially forgot about it, dismissing the technique from my mind as
ludicrous.

Weeks later I had a session with a patient whom I had been treating for
an addictive disorder. She liked pain medications even though she did not
have a pain problem. While we were discussing the various triggers that led
to her desire to use, she began to experience a strong craving for her drug
of choice. I asked her to rate this on a 0 to 10 scale, and she gave it a 10.
That certainly seemed to be an accurate rating, judging by her appearance
at the time. She evidenced tremors and significant changes in her breathing

and facial coloration. I then attempted to assist her in alleviating the craving by taking her through rational emotive imagery, a method that involves altering one's internal talk in order to produce a change in feelings. While this method worked to reduce the craving to a 4, moments later she was able to resurrect the previous 10.

I then recalled the "tapping" article. I explained to the patient that this might seem a bit preposterous, but I wanted her to think about the craving while she tapped under one of her eyes, followed by tapping under one of her arms. I had her do this for a while, going back and forth between the two points, and she then reported a significant reduction in the craving, down to a 4. However, this time a rather interesting thing happened. *Amazing* might be a more accurate descriptor. When I asked her to attempt to bring back the strong craving that she felt before, she was unable to do so. She was unable to resurrect the feelings, even though she thought about the triggers, described the sensations of taking the drug, etc. Both my patient and I were tremendously impressed!

From a more or less scientific point of view, I had to admit that I did not really know what had happened. Was it the tapping itself that produced the result? Was it the fact that the tapping was preceded by rational emotive imagery? Was the patient so profoundly distracted by the tapping that, even when she tried to recall the feelings, she would again return to the tapping in her mind? That is, did we produce some sort of an ongoing distraction that could not be achieved simply by attempting to change what one tells oneself in one's mind? Was this in actuality a placebo effect that would have been produced regardless of where my patient tapped while thinking about the craving? While my mind was filled with all sorts of questions about what actually took place, I realized that I needed to learn more. What would it take to assist the patient in totally alleviating the craving? After all, she was still experiencing craving at a level 4, so, while there was obviously a significant reduction, some craving remained. I felt compelled to investigate this procedure in more detail.

After this seminal event, I decided to learn more about this possibly highly effective and efficient approach for treating addiction. Actually, initially I did not even remember who wrote the "tapping" article, and I could not recall where I had placed it. I looked through the papers at my office and in my study at home, and eventually I found it. The article was written by Roger J. Callahan, Ph.D. I decided to get in touch with him.

Callahan had extensive materials available, including books, self-published papers and manuals, audiotapes, and videotapes. I purchased some of them and began to absorb all of the information I could get my hands on concerning his approach. He and I had many inspiring discussions and he guided me to related literature that was really quite new to me at the time. I read works by orthopedic surgeon Robert O. Becker, radiologist Bjorn Nordenstrom, biologist Rupert Sheldrake, physicist David Bohm, Arthur Young, inventor of the Bell helicopter, Yale researcher Harold Saxon Burr, and others. Of particular interest to me was the field of applied kinesiology, which was developed by George Goodheart, D.C., a highly innovative chiropractor from Detroit, Michigan. I read some of his work as well as that of some of his colleagues, including David S. Walther and John Thie. This eventually led me to investigate related approaches, such as clinical kinesiology (CK), educational kinesiology (Edu-K), Three in One Concepts, acupuncture, acupressure, and reflexology. I also read much of the work of psychiatrist John Diamond, after learning that Callahan partly got his start in this new direction by studying Diamond's applications of kinesiology to emotional problems, what he referred to as behavioral kinesiology. I also had the opportunity to briefly study with Diamond.

Callahan considered much of his work to be proprietary and trade secrets. He had developed a diagnostic system that made it possible for him to determine specifically where the patient needed to tap in order to resolve not only addictive urges but also a wide array of other psychological problems. However, the tuition to learn his diagnostic system was rather steep relative to most other training programs I had attended over the years and, due to concerns about money, as well as my unwillingness to part with so much of it, initially I set out on a course of attempting to "reinvent the wheel," possibly to develop my own energy diagnostic system. Although I succeeded at this task to a large extent, I nonetheless later decided to attend training in the Callahan Techniques™, realizing that knowledge and know-how were more important to me than money. Given all that I have learned and developed since that time, I am grateful that I had the opportunity to study so closely with Roger Callahan.

After completing the seminar on this diagnostic system and working with it for a time, I developed a couple seminars of my own to introduce other professionals to certain aspects of this system — what are referred to as therapeutic recipes or algorithms. My initial training seminar was entitled "Rapidly Resolving Traumatic Memories," and it covered theory, some basic muscle testing to illustrate the interaction between mind and body, and treatments for trauma, specific phobias, anticipatory anxiety, addictive urges, anger, guilt, rage, and psychological reversal. The second seminar in the series was designated "Recipes for Rapid Change," and it expanded the information on psychological reversal and covered a number of additional algorithms and procedures to treat depression, physical pain, obsession, compulsions, panic, agoraphobia, and neurologic disorganization. Since Callahan was beginning to refer to his approach as thought field therapy, the second time I offered these seminars, they were referred to as "Thought Field Therapy Level 1" and "Thought Field Therapy Level 2" respectively. Over time these seminars grew to include increasing amounts of information, and by 1996 the curricula were pretty well established.

By 1998, I discontinued offering TFT Level 1 and TFT Level 2 seminars on a regular basis and instead placed the information contained in those two seminars in one manual and began offering a seminar referred to as "Thought Field Therapy Combined." By this time I had decided to simply give participants all of the information on algorithms "up front," take them through examples and demonstrations of the treatment process, and then send them off to practice in the privacy of their own personal workshops, their private and public practices. After that I developed a training program entitled *The New Energy Psychology*, a term that more accurately reflected the curricula, since it entailed a wider coverage of energy psychotherapy, TFT being an aspect of that field of endeavor.

Stepping back a bit, in 1995, at the request of Charles Figley, Ph.D., I wrote a couple of articles for the *Electronic Journal of Traumatology*: "Reflections on Active Ingredients in Efficient Treatments of PTSD," Parts 1 and 2, which attempted to explore some relatively new and highly efficient psychotherapeutic approaches, including thought field therapy, and to glean some of the active ingredients that account for their effectiveness and efficiency. Some time in 1996, I was again contacted by Charles, who asked me if I wanted to write a book. I recall saying, "I thought you'd never ask!" Over the next year and a half I wrote *Energy Psychology: Explorations at the Interface of Energy, Cognition, Behavior, and Health* (1998, CRC Press). That book introduced the fields of psychology and psychotherapy to what I envisioned as a new field of research and practice. Although bioenergy ideas had been around for quite a while (about 7,000 years), for the most part these were relatively new concepts to psychology and psychotherapy, since little Western empirical research had been conducted in this area, and most psychotherapists were not utilizing bioenergetic understanding in their practices.

About a year prior to the publication of *Energy Psychology*, I began to present "Energy Diagnostic and Treatment Methods" (EDxTM), the system that is the subject of the present book. This methodology is an extension of the one I developed prior to studying with Callahan and is also the result of several serendipitous findings that, in my experience, considerably improve upon previous work in this area. After having published a case study on TFT in *The Family Therapy Networker* entitled "A No-Talk Cure for Trauma: Thought Field Therapy Seems to Violate All the Rules" (1997a), I was contacted by Susan Munro of W. W. Norton, who asked me if I would like to write a book on my diagnostic system. So here we are.

What has interested me greatly about bioenergetic approaches to psychotherapy is my experience of their effectiveness and efficiency, as well as the fact that the approach is so dramatically distinct from other approaches to therapy. While most psychotherapeutic approaches prove beneficial to varying degrees, depending upon the person and condition being treated, I had never before found an approach to be so singularly rapid in its effects. Not only has my clinical experience confirmed this, but I have also had many personal experiences in support of those findings.

While I was studying thought field therapy, I was also investigating eye movement desensitization and reprocessing (Shapiro, 1995).[1] During a small group exercise at an EMDR conference, I was able to resolve a traumatic incident from my past with the assistance of a colleague. The trauma concerned an incident from when I was approximately 11 years of age. My mother died of cancer when I was 12, and there were many events preceding and after her death that bothered me, regardless of the fact that I was in my mid-forties at the time of the seminar.

The memory treated at that conference was a moment in time when my father had returned from the hospital with my mother. I was upstairs making my younger brothers' beds and my father entered the room, announcing that he wanted to talk to me about something. I recall telling him that I understood that Mom was sick, and that I needed to help out around the house, and that I was doing just that. I imagine that he had to remind me many times to help out, since that was the first thing that occurred to me when he said we needed to talk. Maybe I also sensed something about what he was going to tell me, but I do not recall that for certain. But I vividly

---

[1] Although distinct in many respects, eye movement desensitization and reprocessing (EMDR) has similarities to rapid eye technology (Johnson, 1994) and eye movement integration (Andreas & Andreas, 1995).

remember him saying, "No, that's not what I need to talk to you about. We just came from the doctor."

He hesitated and I asked him what the doctor had to say, likely bracing myself for the news. "The doctor said that Mom is going to die." At that moment it felt like a high voltage of electricity passing through my body, followed by my feeling numb and dazed by what I had just been told. I remember feeling very weak at the moment but then I stood up slowly and started to walk out of the room, practically zombie-like. Then I turned around, ran to my father, and cried deeply. He told me that I needed to be strong and that I could not let my mother see me like this.

After he left the room, it took quite a while for me to regain my composure. I made several attempts to descend the stairs to the kitchen to visit with my mother. In one instance I remember hearing her talking about some cookies she was eating while drinking coffee at the kitchen table. They were waffle cookies, what we called pizelles. I heard her say, "I love these cookies." I remember that that comment stirred up a lot of tears for me, as I thought that she would not be able to enjoy them for long since she was going to die. I had to run upstairs again in an effort to regain my composure. When I finally made it downstairs she asked me if I had been crying, and I offered her some feeble excuse, that I had a cold or a headache.

That was the memory. Recalling the part where my father told me about the inevitable during EMDR, the severe distress was dissolved. It has remained with me a sacred memory with some sorrow, but the distress is gone. I imagine that even the remaining sorrow could be eliminated, but I've chosen not to do that.

There were, of course, many other painful memories around the death of my mother. She had cancer for well over a year, suffering in bed — lots of time for me to accumulate pain and despair. And there were many other unhappy memories really branded in my mind and heart about the later death of my father and two younger brothers, a distressing divorce, and more. But they were not merely painful memories; the traumas also affected my life as a whole in many respects. I had tried many times in the past to resolve the distress by discussing the events, emotionally reliving them, and using various techniques that I had learned. Through TFT and related methods that I have discovered through experimentation, I have been able to resolve massive amounts of personal distress, without having to experience abreaction along the way. The memories remain, but the severe pain is gone. Gratifyingly, I have found that I can also consistently assist others in these ways as well. And the relief is not simply related to trauma, although trauma does seem to figure into a wide range of problems. These methods are also helpful in the treatment of various affect and behavioral problems, including depression, anxiety-based conditions, addiction, anger, rage, jealousy, guilt, self-esteem issues, and so on.[2]

This book is about the application of diagnostic and treatment methods rooted in an energy paradigm. In many respects it is a manual that guides the motivated practitioner and researcher through a variety of protocols to determine the energetic structure of a psychological problem and to apply treatments that emanate from this causal diagnosis. This is not about diagnosis in a nosological sense, but rather about diagnosis resulting from an analysis of the energy configuration at the basis of the condition. Surely there is an interrelationship here, but this approach is radically distinct from standard psychiatric nosology.

The chapters have been arranged in order of importance. For the most part one must understand the earlier chapters if the later ones are to be adequately understood and absorbed. Additionally, for the convenience of the reader, I have been intentionally redundant when delineating certain protocols, so as to avoid as much as possible having to turn back and forth between chapters.

A brief summary of some of the highlights of each chapter follows:

Chapter 1 covers a number of the assumptions in psychological science and those specifically related to energy diagnostic and treatment methods. Also covered are *qi*, the multifaceted "energy" of meridian approaches such as acupuncture; various acupoints such as alarm, sedation, and tonification points; acupoint stimulation by tapping, pressure, and intention; applied kinesiology; manual muscle testing; therapy localization; attunement; disruptions in the body's energy system as related to psychological problems; energy balancing; resonance locking methods; and intentionality.

Chapter 2 covers client preparation and debriefing issues. While diagnosing and balancing the bioenergy system is the principal methodology offered in this text, it is best conducted within a solid therapeutic relationship. With this in mind, the chapter covers issues such as rapport, empathy, pacing and

---

[2]The question may arise in the reader's mind that if EMDR is so effective in alleviating posttraumatic stress, why do anything else? As effective as EMDR is, it occasionally results in abreaction, which requires considerable skill to handle in a therapeutically beneficial manner. Additionally, the approach described here has a wider range of applicability than many other methods. I would like to point out, however, that I especially appreciate the attention Shapiro (1995) has given to installing positive cognition, which is incorporated into the methods presented in this book.

leading, expectations, explaining the method, client commitment, permission, the client-therapist partnership, attunement and exposure, measurement of treatment results, client skepticism, aspects and holons, energy toxins, and thought awareness.

Chapter 3 provides details on the application of manual muscle testing in the diagnosis and treatment of psychological problems. While manual muscle testing can be a fairly simple and straightforward procedure, instances arise when greater skill is needed. There are a number of variables that the highly skilled examiner is aware of and prepared to address efficiently when necessary. This chapter attempts to cover many of those variables and related procedures.

Chapter 4 addresses the diagnosis and treatment of neurologic disorganization. This condition is singularly relevant, since it is often consistent with physical awkwardness, difficulties with coordination, problems with directionality, and learning difficulties. It may also impede therapeutic progress. When neurologic disorganization is present it is impossible to accurately calibrate muscle response, hindering energy diagnostics.

Chapter 5 provides in-depth coverage of the various facets of psychological reversal, significant blocks to treatment effectiveness. The reader is provided with details on how to apply manual muscle testing to diagnose and correct for massive/global, specific, mini/intervening, and criteria-related reversals.

Chapter 6 focuses on distinctions among three energy treatment approaches: behavioral kinesiology (Diamond, 1978, 1979, 1980a, 1980b, 1985), thought field therapy (Callahan, 1985; Callahan & Callahan, 1996), and the methodology presented in this book, referred to as energy diagnostic and treatment methods or EDxTM (Gallo, 1997b). Also covered are the methodology and rationale of procedures such as the nine gamut treatments, brain balancing procedure, cross-crawl exercises, as well as rapid stress reduction techniques, including the floor-to-ceiling eye roll and the elaborated eye roll.

Chapter 7 introduces a couple of global treatment protocols that have been found to be effective for a wide range of clinical problems. Using these therapeutic recipes can be considered a first step toward developing expertise with energy diagnostic and treatment methods. These procedures can be regularly incorporated into various phases of the overall treatment regime. They can also be utilized easily by clients for maintenance, self-treatment between sessions, and other problems that may arise after formal treatment has been completed.

Chapter 8, by way of description and pictures, specifies the various test and treatment points employed in the diagnosis and treatment of the bioenergy aspects of psychological disturbances. The reader is assisted in precisely locating the alarm or test points used to diagnose meridian imbalance, as well as preferred treatment points used to further evaluate and alleviate imbalance within the energy system.

Chapter 9 covers the most basic diagnostic-treatment protocol, what is referred to as single-point protocol. The guiding assumption of this protocol is that the energy disruptions at the basis of a psychological problem can be efficiently treated by addressing one acupoint at a time. The protocol entails locating a single treatment point and then having the client physically tap or percuss on that point in order to stimulate the energy system and thus remove the negative affects or emotions associated with the psychological problem. Here it is assumed that the single point is the principal meridian point involved in the energy disruption. Even though other meridians and associated acupoints may be involved in a condition, treatment of the nodal point will efficiently reverberate and neutralize the problem. Theoretically, there is assumed to be an affect-perturbation connection, so that stimulating the energy system at a specific locale serves to collapse or subsume the perturbations in the thought field germane to the psychological problem.

Chapter 9 also covers the multi-point protocol or constellation elaboration. This protocol is indicated when the single-point protocol does not achieve sufficient results for the client. The guiding assumption is that the energy disruptions at the basis of a psychological problem can be treated by addressing a cluster of acupoints at the same time. The protocol entails locating several simultaneously active points and then having the client physically tap or percuss on those points in order to stimulate the energy system and thus remove the negative affects or emotions associated with the psychological problem.

Chapter 10 introduces the application of manual muscle testing in the diagnosis and treatment of negative core beliefs. Pragmatically the core beliefs protocol is employed when the single-point and multi-point protocols do not achieve adequate results or when it is obvious that the client's clinical condition and/or belief structure is interfering with achieving appreciable results. The guiding assumption of this protocol is that the energy disruptions at the basis of a psychological problem can be more substantially treated by addressing the energy structure of the underlying core belief or beliefs.

While many patients can be assisted by employing global treatments, single-point or multi-point protocols, with some requiring primary or attendant treatment of various dysfunctional core beliefs, still others will evidence a recalcitrant tendency for the primary symptoms to be resurrected or to resist treatment efforts altogether. In many such instances, an exogenous substance is the culprit. Chapter 11 provides detailed procedures for the diagnosis, management, and treatment of energy toxins.

With Chapter 12, the book comes to a close, touching on issues of paradigms, kinesiology, research, ethics, and the future of energy psychology.

Now it is time to fill in the blanks. I ask only that you keep an open mind and maintain a spirit of experimentation and adventure as you absorb what follows. I appreciate your willingness to pursue the diligent study required to integrate these protocols into your work. With practice you will find this information enlightening, beneficial to yourself and your patients, and also of heuristic value. I trust that as you come to appreciate the relevance of this approach, you will pursue more study and eventually advance the field further than I have.

Energy Diagnostic and Treatment Methods

Chapter 1

ASSUMPTIONS AND ROOTS

As a first approximation, I define "belief" not as the object of believing (a dogma, a program, etc.) but as the subject's investment in a proposition, the act of saying it and considering it as true.

—*Michel de Certeau*, The Practice of Everyday Life

THERE IS A TALE about a philosopher of science who was lecturing on the role of assumptions in the development of knowledge. He noted that our presuppositions, upon which knowledge is pursued, rest upon little more than our willingness to have faith in them. As an illustrative analogy he offered that the planets revolve around the sun, supported by nothing other than our assumptions or theories about something we call *gravity*.

When the lecture was over, an elderly gentleman approached the philosopher, expressing enthusiasm about the presentation but also saying that he begged to disagree about the orbiting planets. He insisted instead that the planets actually rest on the backs of giant tortoises that walk around the sun along the paths we call orbits.

In an effort to enlighten the old man further regarding the true purpose of the analogy, the philosopher simply inquired as to what might be supporting the creatures as they make their trek around the sun.

To this the man quickly and adamantly replied, "Oh, no, sir! You ain't gonna get me on that one. It's turtles all the way down!"

But of course it cannot be "turtles all the way down." There has to be a point at which we run out of turtles, where our presuppositions become starkly epistemologically evident. So we begin our discussion with a number of assumptions for which there is some rational, intuitive, or clinical support. But like all assumptions, in reality they merely represent the base or foundation upon which an edifice is constructed, their true value being realized in terms of the power and stability of the structures upon which they rest. Necessarily, all structures eventually topple more or less, as their foundations can only support so much. Thus, in the area of physics, for example, Newtonian conceptualizations or laws make sense and accurate predictions within a delimited realm, but necessitate notable adjustments when making calculations concerning subatomic particles (or are "they" waves?), velocities approaching the speed of light (assumed to be the ultimate speed), travel between point A and point B (or is it all of a sudden?), and so forth.

ASSUMPTIONS OF PSYCHOLOGICAL SCIENCE

With regard to psychological functioning and dysfunction, there are a variety of theoretical models or frameworks that attempt to explain and make predictions, with psychotherapies and other kinds of interventions resting upon them. For instance, we can punctuate psychological disturbances as manifestations of unconscious dynamics, cognitive schemas, schedules of reinforcement and conditioning, systemic interactions, maladies of brain structures and neurochemistry, heredity, and so on. We assume that all of these facets and conceptualizations are relevant and valid to a greater or lesser extent, depending upon the condition under consideration. Therefore, while autism certainly entails neurological, behavioral, systemic, and cognitive components, the degree of causality attributed to each will vary. If we were to focus solely on the interactions within the family as the cause, to the neglect of neurological and behavioral dimensions, our ability to intercede would be greatly limited. So, too, if we were to consider depression as if it were solely a chemical imbalance, without attending to the individual's life circumstances and the cognitive, behavioral, and energetic aspects of the condition, we would be limited in our ability to assist the client in achieving ongoing relief. Many reductionistic models reach their limits of applicability quickly. We are in search of a universal field theory of mind that will allow us to determine precisely which aspects of functioning are most relevant when.

BIOENERGY ASSUMPTIONS

Here we offer an assumption that is generally seen as being somewhat off the beaten path: that *subtle bioenergy* exists. While there is some evidence for the existence of subtle energy fields (Becker, 1990; Becker, Reichmanis, & Marino, 1976; Becker & Selden, 1985; Burr, 1972; Gallo, 1998; Gerber,

1988; Nordenstrom, 1983; Sheldrake, 1981), this is hardly universally accepted. Pomeranz (1996) points out that, while his research has convinced him that acupuncture is effective beyond any placebo effect, he has found no convincing evidence for the existence of *qi*, the subtle energy that acupuncture is supposed to regulate.

With these cautions in mind, it is proposed that psychological functioning in general and psychological disturbances in particular can be effectively punctuated, to a significant degree, in terms of subtle bioenergy information or configurations.[1] Healthy psychological functioning, as well as health in general, is assumed to be consistent with a balance or unobstructed current of bioenergy, while psychological disturbances are consistent with imbalance or encumbered "flow." In a related sense, healthy as compared to diseased psychological functioning may be described otherwise in terms of bioenergy vibrations (Gerber, 1988). Thus, the existence of subtle bioenergy and specific characteristics within this dimension becomes one of our fundamental assumptions. These same bioenergy attributes are described throughout the acupuncture and meridian literature. The bioenergy has been referred to by such terms as the Chinese *chi* or *qi* (pronounced *chee*), the Japanese *ki* (pronounced *key*), the Indian *prana*, life energy, Paracelsus's *archaeus*, Hypocrites's *vis medicatrix naturae*, and more.

Qi

The idea of qi does not fit neatly into one delimited scientific definition. Qi is not equivalent to what Westerners have in mind when referring to energy, for as used in traditional Chinese medicine, qi is a much more encompassing and versatile aspect of being (Zmiewski, Wiseman, & Ellis, 1985). According to some researchers, qi or bioenergy is largely electrical (Becker, 1990; Becker & Selden, 1985), while others think of qi as magnetic, thermal, light, acoustical, etc.[2]

---

[1]While energy psychology can be seen as solely attending to subtle bioenergy, I believe that there is a cybernetic interface among energy, thought, cognition, neurology, chemistry, behavior, and health.

[2]Further, traditional Chinese medicine recognizes a variety of qi, including *tian qi* (sky or universe), *di qi* (earth), and *ren qi* (human), not to mention plant qi and animal qi. Electrical energy is designated as *dian qi*, whereas heat is referred to as *re qi*. When a being is alive, the vital energy is called *huo qi*. At death the dead qi is called *si qi*. When a person is functioning to his or her spiritual best, the energy is *zheng qi* (Yang, 1989). Qi can also be translated as mind, power, and influence.

Biofields

To a large extent qi or bioenergy also speaks of fields, which may be referred to as *biofields* (Gallo, 1998). There are two diametrically opposed views of biofields: One states that biofields are epiphenomena of the physical body; the other that they account for the physical body in addition to its idiosyncratic forms. It is well known that every atom that makes up the material body is replaced in its entirety approximately every four to seven years. What accounts for the replication and maintenance of form? It is also well known that every cell of an organism contains the genetic makeup of the entire body. But how does a hand know to be a hand, a foot to be a foot, the brain to differentiate from tendon and bone? Is this merely the result of chemical reactions? Or is there an energy, an influence, a forming principle directing the show, catalyzing the process of growth, indeed replicating the form? This is consistent with Sheldrake's notions of *morphogenetic fields, morphic resonance*, and the *hypothesis of formative causation* (1981) as well as Burr's findings concerning *life fields* or *L fields* (1972).

In the realm of psychological functioning or mind, are psychological disturbances merely a function of conditioning history? Or is their presence evidence of anomalous DNA and/or "chemical imbalance"? Is the neurologic hardware wired incorrectly, scarred, or diseased? Is the person plagued by an affliction of incorrect thinking, to which we might offer a course in formal logic, provide a reframe, spin a paradox or two, possibly encourage a paradigmatic shift toward consciousness of thought and mind?

It is suggested that all of these avenues are simultaneously correct to varying degrees, for we are surely able to punctuate the plethora of data available to our senses and to our instruments in a variety of ways, attempting to make sense of the elephant who one day strolled into our blind midst. The psychological disturbances we observe are at once environmental-behavioral, systemic, cognitive, precognitive, neurologic, chemical, and, I add rather emphatically, *bioenergetic*! Some conditions may be defined as predominantly one or another, but certainly all aspects come into play to some extent. And since energy is the most fundamental aspect of our material reality, in a sense it is invariably central, most fundamentally causal, although it is conceivable that *consciousness* (Goswami, 1993) and *action* (Young, 1976a, 1976b, 1984) are more fundamental yet, albeit intertwined with energy and fields. The *fundamentality* of consciousness and action can be recognized, in that even light is observed to travel with a certain rationality that suggests it is somehow conscious and volitional in its pursuit. In this regard, note findings in the area of quantum physics, such as the double-slit experiments suggesting that photons make choices (Zukav, 1979).

Meridians

Even though the longevity of an idea does not prove its validity, it may be assumed that since acupuncture and related meridian therapies have been in existence for perhaps as long as 5,000 years, there is at least some validity to the idea of meridians or energy channels. The meridians have been described in the literature dating back to the *Nei Jing* (also called *Nei Ching*),[3] the first text on internal medicine, prepared during the reign of Huang Ti, the Yellow Emperor of China (2690–2590 BC). Judging by the fact that before and during that period knowledge was generally communicated in oral and practicum forms, the information upon which the *Nei Jing* is based is likely far more ancient than the texts themselves.

As much as a couple millennia preceding the Chinese discovery, a similar finding was made in India. There are also indications that comparable discoveries occurred throughout the world, including Europe, Egypt, Arabia, Brazil, among the Bantu tribes of Africa, and the Eskimos. Goodheart (1987) points out that "[t]he papyrus ebers of 1150 BC, one of the most important of the ancient Egyptian medical treatises, refers to a book on the subject of muscles which would correspond to the 12 [primary] meridians of acupuncture" (p. 10).

There is also some empirical support for the existence of meridians (Becker, 1990; Becker, Reichmanis, & Marino, 1976; Becker & Selden, 1985; de Vernejoul, Albarède, & Darras, 1985). Thus, it is proposed that there are twelve primary meridians, most of which pass through a number of bodily organs for which they are named: *lung, large intestine, stomach, spleen,[4] small intestine, bladder, pericardium,[5] kidney, heart, triple ener-*

---

[3]*Nei* translates as *internal*. *Jing* or *ching* can be defined variably, depending if it is used as a noun, verb, or adjective (Yang, 1989). In this context it appears to mean *essence*. Thus *Nei Jing* refers to *internal essence*. *Jing* is the essence of *qi* (energy) and *shen* (spirit).

[4]The spleen meridian has also been referred to as the pancreas meridian. However, we are employing the *Standard International Nomenclature* for the twelve primary and the collector meridians addressed in the system covered in this text.

[5]The pericardium meridian has also been referred to as the circulation sex meridian.

gizer,[6] *gall bladder,* and *liver.*[7] Additionally, there are eight extraordinary vessels, also referred to as collector meridians, the two most significant of which are the *governing vessel,* which begins below the coccyx and extends to the upper lip; and the *conception vessel,* which begins at the perineum and ends at the lower lip. The remaining extraordinary vessels are designated as follows: *thrusting, girdle, yang heel, yin heel, yang linking,* and *yin linking* (Yang, 1989).[8] In a sense there is only one meridian, in that the meridians connect one into the other; however, there is evidence that each of the demarcations along the path has some specificity in terms of function.

Acupoints

Similarly, we may also assume that many of the acupoints, depending upon their location on the meridians, have distinct functions, perhaps accounting for unique vibrations or energy frequencies as well as neurologic specificity. At some locations the distinction is rather pronounced, and at other locations there is a mere nuance of difference. This is consistent with the literature on acupuncture, which describes a rich variety of individual points. *Alarm points,* which are employed in a number of systems, are utilized for diagnosis and treatment. *Akabane points,* on fingernails and toenails, also referred to as entrance and exit points of meridians, are used to transmit energy between meridians. *Horary points* become active during specific two-hour time frames and are relevant with respect to the *five elements theory* of acupuncture. *Hsi points* (pronounced *she*) are used to "turbo charge" meridians that are extremely deficient in energy. *Luo points* (pronounced *low*) balance energy between bilateral equivalent meridians. *Sedation points* are employed to balance overactive meridians, while *tonification points* balance underactive meridians. *Source points* affect the entire meridian (Walther, 1988). While each of these points appears to affect the balance within and between the meridians in distinct ways, they have other characteristics as well. According to the model being presented here, not only is each meridian associated

------

[6]The triple energizer meridian, also referred to by terms such as triple heater and triple warmer, does not exist as an anatomical organ in modern anatomy.

[7]There is some uncertainty about the degree of correlation between the names Western medicine has given to certain organs and the ancient Chinese designations. In traditional Chinese medicine, for example, the "spleen" is involved with digestion and the "kidney" is related to the genitals (Gunn, 1998).

[8]This volume attends only to the conception and governing vessels.

with specific muscles (Goodheart, 1987; Thie, 1973) and specific emotions (Diamond, 1985), but various points along the meridians also carry distinct emotional/issue nuances.[9] (See Chapter 8 for locations of acupoints employed in this system.)

Acupoint Stimulation

The acupoints can be stimulated in a variety of ways to affect the balance or homeostasis within the energy system. Acupuncture needles and manual pressure or acupressure[10] are the most commonly known means. However, stimulation of acupoints can also be produced by burning moxi, an herb, on the acupoint; by creating a vacuum at the location of a relevant point; by electricity, magnets, cold laser, ultrasound, other types of sound, "liquid needle," tapping, etc. The meridian(s) as a whole may also be balanced in other ways, such as by manually tracing in the direction of meridian flow, hatha yoga exercises, meditation, adjusting muscles, affirmations, music, etc. We shall be focusing primarily on the utility of pressure or percussing (i.e., tapping) on meridian points in order to stimulate the flow of bioenergy and thus alleviate psychological disturbances; however, we shall also look at the relevance of affirmations (Diamond, 1985) and intentionality (Tiller, 1997) with respect to the movement and balancing of energy.

Manual Indicator Muscle Testing

Although the topic of manual muscle testing is expanded upon in later chapters, let me briefly mention various assumptions in this area. I propose that *indicator muscle* testing is reflective of specific information within thought fields when a psychological problem is attuned, assuming that the test is being properly conducted at the time.[11] Proper utilization of the test

---

[9] The meridians are also associated with organs, as their names suggest; however, since the ancient Chinese knew little about internal anatomy, the names attributed to the meridians corresponded to physiological functions on the basis of their observations and were not limited to specific organs. Therefore, the meridian-organ connection is not always in agreement with our scientific understanding (Beyens, 1998).

[10] Acupressure is a misnomer since it literally means needle (i.e., *acu*) pressure. The Japanese shiatsu, which is essentially equivalent to acupressure, is a more accurate term, since it roughly translates as "treatment by finger pressure."

[11] "When a muscle not known to be associated with a reflex or other factor is used to evaluate therapy localization, it is called an indicator muscle" (Walther, 1988, p. 38).

precludes conscious or subconscious confounding on the part of the tester and/or subject, physiologic problems with the muscle being challenged, and other confounding variables. Additionally, it is clear that a muscle test is simply that, a *test*, which obviously entails issues of reliability and validity. In the present context, the purpose of the test is to acquire information about what treatment is needed in order to alleviate the psychological problem. The ultimate verification of the test is found in the outcome obtained, namely, alleviation of the targeted problem. Therefore, the test is employed as an indicator. In this regard, if a muscle test were to indicate that treating a specific meridian was needed to alleviate a disturbance, we would not simply accept the test as the final authority. We would await the outcome. If the outcome were positive, we would be inclined to conclude that the test was accurate, that it correlated perfectly or nearly perfectly with treatment needs. If, on the other hand, the problem were not alleviated, we might be inclined to question the validity of the test in that particular context. While some other factor might be involved, we would nonetheless scrutinize the test results.

Meridian Diagnosis: Pulse Testing

Imbalance within the energy system, and specifically within and between meridians, can be diagnosed in several ways. Probably the most complex method involves assessment of twelve pulses located on the wrists on the radial artery at the palmer thumb side, six on each wrist (see Figure 1.1). The acupuncturist skilled in this method places a finger at the location of each of the various pulses that correlate with the meridians and is reportedly able to feel the differences with respect to energy within the meridian, this

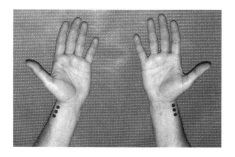

Figure 1.1 Meridian wrist pulses

being determined by the relative strength and other qualities of the various pulses. According to most systems, light touch on the left wrist, with increasing distance from the thumb, localizes *small intestine, gall bladder,* and *bladder,* whereas deep touch on the left wrist indicates *heart, liver,* and *kidney* with increasing distance from the thumb. Light touch on the right wrist, with increasing distance from the thumb, localizes *large intestine, stomach,* and *triple-energizer,* and deep touch on the right wrist indicates *lung, spleen,* and *pericardium* with increasing distance from the thumb. Distinctions among these pulses inform the acupuncturist as to which meridian(s) require therapeutic attention. Obviously, it takes extensive practice and years of experience to develop the sensitivity to conduct this test proficiently. To complicate matters further, it should be noted that there are many different and highly complex pulse diagnosis systems, and the diagnostic conclusions reached as a result of each can vary widely (Gunn, 1998). Therefore this approach to diagnosis becomes rather cumbersome and not readily utilized by the psychotherapy practitioner.

Meridian Diagnosis: Pulse-Indicator Muscle Testing

The labor involved in developing tactile sensitivity to the pulses can sometimes be circumvented by touching or therapy localizing the pulses while testing an indicator muscle (Stokes & Whiteside, 1981). The examiner begins by checking three pulses simultaneously by placing three fingers of one hand at the location of the pulses, first with light touch and then with deep touch, each time testing a strong indicator muscle (IM), perhaps the middle deltoid, in which case the opposite arm is extended at right angle to the side.[12] Let us say that the examiner is testing the left wrist pulses. Remember, light touch designates *small intestine, gall bladder,* and *bladder,* with increasing distance from the subject's thumb. If the muscle weakens while the examiner simultaneously touches all three pulses with the light touch, it is concluded that at least one of the pulses (i.e., meridians) accounts for the muscle weakness. The examiner next touches each individual pulse lightly, until the IM weakens again at a specific location, perhaps the bladder pulse.

---

[12]An indicator muscle (IM) is any intact muscle that can be used in conjunction with therapy localization (TL) to assess meridian functioning as well as other bodily functions. TL involves either the tester or subject touching specific locations on the body while the IM is challenged, thus revealing important information about functions related to the point touched.

This reveals a disruption within the bladder meridian, which would then be the target of therapeutic attention. Alternatively, the subject can touch the pulses while the examiner challenges an indicator muscle. In this instance a muscle such as the quadriceps might be challenged.

Alarm Point Testing

An important feature of our method is the use of *alarm points*. This involves testing an indicator muscle while having the subject touch each of the alarm points. If a subject consciously brings to mind or otherwise accesses an issue involving emotional distress during the testing, the alarm point that produces a change in muscle response (i.e., generally a change from relatively *weak* to relatively *strong*) is the point associated with the meridian(s) most fundamentally involved in the emotional disturbance. One feasible interpretation of this phenomenon is that touching the alarm point serves to complete or close a circuit that is responsible for or correlated with the negative psychological response. Alternatively, it might be discussed or framed in terms of a communication from the body, or perhaps from the unconscious, indicating the meridian that needs therapeutic attention. In either respect, energy disruption is equivalent to emotional disturbance.

Perturbations

It should be noted that, in addition to disruptions within a meridian, something else must be occurring when a "negative" emotion or other undesired "expression" appears. The fact that a specific thought or awareness results in an energy meridian imbalance indicates that the thought itself must in some way cause the imbalance. The connection between thoughts and emotions is well established in my experience. Perhaps it can be concluded that the thought contains a trigger of sorts that catalyzes the disruption within the meridian. In this sense we might conclude that the thought holds within it or has attached to it an electromagnetic, photoelectric, or other energetic marker that initiates or generates the imbalance. Roger Callahan coined the term *perturbation* (p) for these features or energetic codes contained within the thought. While thoughts entail neurologic, chemical, and cognitive aspects, additionally they are inextricably bound in fields, and thus the term *thought field* (*tf*) appears to be most appropriate and accurate (Callahan & Callahan, 1996).

A distinction worth noting is that the perturbation is designated as such because it causes a disruption in the state of harmony or balance that is considered to be the normal or healthy state of affairs.[13] Tapping on meridian points is hypothesized by the original theory to collapse or subsume the perturbations in the thought field by mobilizing the subtle energy system in distinct sectors (i.e., meridians). An alternative interpretation, which appears to be revealing in other respects and perhaps more palatable across the natural sciences, is that stimulating the energy system in this manner actually introduces perturbations into the field, thereby disrupting the stability of the "pathologic" thought field. The thought field, like any field, exists as a pattern or form with certain degrees of stability or homeostasis. The goal of intervention is to profoundly alter the integrity of such pathognomonic energy fields at sufficiently relevant levels, so that a return to the previous forms becomes less probable or even impossible. Thus, in one sense the goal of therapy is to introduce perturbations rather than to simply remove them, although the perturbations introduced are intended to remove those that disrupt homeostasis.

Therapy Localization

Manual muscle testing and therapy localization are integrally related. Albeit more versatile in its applications, the muscle response is analogous to a biofeedback monitor that provides information about specific functions.

> A major development in applied kinesiology occurred when Goodheart observed that if a client touched an area of dysfunction, the results of manual muscle testing changed. A muscle that previously tested weak became strong when the client touched the area of dysfunction. The system is called therapy localization (TL). It finds the location of a problem, but it does not necessarily tell you **what** is wrong. (Walther, 1988, p. 37)

When therapy localizing with respect to a specific perturbed thought field (i.e., a psychological disturbance or issue), the examiner initially tests a strong intact indicator muscle *in the clear*, which means that the subject is

---

[13] Perturb is from the Latin *pertubare* [*per* (to or toward) + *tubare* (confusion)] meaning to throw into confusion or disorder.

not accessing a disturbing thought or the psychological issue, touching anyplace on his or her body, or touching anything else for that matter. This phase provides a baseline or pretest.

After testing *in the clear*, the subject is asked to think of the psychological issue (e.g., trauma, phobia, relationship problem), and then the indicator muscle is again tested. At this point a change in muscle response is generally observed, usually a detectable weakening of the muscle response. Thus, before and after measures have been obtained. It is assumed that this change in muscle response is relevant to the psychological issue at hand. Here we are observing an important connection between mind and body, similar to that evident when one is presented with shocking news, a felt and often quite visible weakness. For example, how many of us have experienced feeling faint or our legs weakening upon learning of the death of a loved one or some other tragedy? The awareness of the situation or event in thought affects one's energy system, and therefore the physical body.

With regard to the weakening indicator muscle, at this point the question becomes, "What will now cause the muscle to test strong?" Whatever causes the muscle to reestablish its strength is the *royal road to cure*. While a multitude of effective therapeutic options exist for any particular problem, this method makes it possible to address individual differences and precisely define the person's therapeutic needs. Rather than employing the same therapy with everyone who has a "specific" problem, such as "depression," therapy localization makes it possible to more accurately diagnose the problem and provide relevant treatments. Therefore this approach is truly a causal diagnostic-therapeutic method.

While there are many options available with this overall approach, one highly versatile method, touched on earlier, involves therapy localizing meridian alarm points in order to determine the bioenergy aspects of the psychological issue. For example, if while the client thinks of the disturbing thought, the muscle weakness is alleviated after she/he touches the alarm point for the stomach meridian and not when she/he touches the alarm point for the kidney meridian, we can conclude that the bioenergy disruption is located within the stomach meridian rather than the kidney meridian. It now becomes simply a matter of more precisely mapping the origin within the disturbed meridian, this again being discerned by having the subject or therapist touch various acupoints along the involved meridian until a point is disclosed that cancels out the muscle weakness. This may be any relevant point along the stomach meridian, such as stomach-1, stomach-4, stomach-

12, etc. Thus if ST-1 tests strong, stimulating that point along the stomach meridian is likely to help in alleviating the psychological disturbance.

Although in most instances the examiner will locate a strong indicator muscle that weakens in response to the psychological issue, and then attempt to locate an alarm point that alleviates the weak response, this is merely one side of the diagnostic coin, what has been referred to as *double negative testing* (Diamond, 1985). At times the psychological issue will not result in a weakening response, but the muscle will remain firm.[14] In such instances, assuming that the psychological issue is attuned, the examiner need only pursue the test point that cancels out the strong muscle response in order to diagnose the therapeutic needs. As a corollary to this, it should be borne in mind that, once treatment has alleviated the weak muscle response in the case of double negative testing, therapy localizing the previously revealing alarm point should not result in a weakening of the indicator muscle, unless disruption continues within that sector of the energy system.

Meridians and Emotions

There appears to be an interface between meridians and emotions, such that various positive emotions are evident when the meridians are balanced (e.g., love, joy, cheer, forgiveness, tranquillity) and various negative emotions predominate when the meridians are disrupted (e.g., hate, sadness, unhappiness, anger, disgust). Some have reported an association between specific meridians and specific emotions. In this regard, although there is one continuous, interconnected bioenergy system, the system is nonetheless divided into segments or meridians, and within each of the meridians are acupoints that serve as *booster amplifiers* (Becker & Selden, 1985). The meridians have been correlated with organs, muscles, and emotions. However, there is no consensus as to which emotions are "housed" within which meridians. For example, in Table 1.1, note the variations regarding negative emotional designations from Diamond (1985), Durlacher (1994), Teeguarden (1996), and Whisenant (1990).

Diamond (personal communication, 1997) asserts that he arrived at his designations by way of manual muscle testing. However, Whisenant (1990),

---

[14]While this may be consistent with psychological reversal (see Chapter 5), this is not invariably the case.

Table 1.1

Meridians and Associated Emotions According to Various Investigators

MERIDIAN	DIAMOND	DURLACHER	TEEGUARDEN	WHISENANT
Stomach	Disgust Deprivation Nausea	Disgust	Anxiety Reclusive	Depression Obsession Pensiveness
Spleen	Anxiety	Low self-esteem	Overconcern Worry	Pensiveness Overconcern Worry
Bladder	Restlessness Frustration Impatience	Miffed	Fear of feelings Desire to escape	Fear Tension Caution
Heart	Anger	Overjoyed	Overexcitement Shock	Overexcitement

who also employed manual muscle testing to correlate meridians and emo-tions, reports diverse designations. Among other possibilities, it is likely that these differences are a function of sampling error and acupoint distinctions.

My hunch is that there are finer distinctions to be made, and that different acupoints along each meridian correlate with different emotions and emo-tional nuances. While research is needed to shed more light on this hypothe-sis, at the present time there does seem to be consistency within individual subjects evaluated in this manner. That is, such a correlation has been suggested as a result of my evaluating a wide array of subjects via manual muscle testing and other clinical observations. Even if future research does not confirm a universal specific meridian/specific emotion or specific acu-point/specific emotion relationship, relatively little will be lost from the standpoint of therapeutic intervention. For diagnostic purposes, the relevant factor is the location of the energy disruption, regardless of what emotion is correlated with it.

Attunement

In order for the energetic aspects of a specific psychological problem to be deciphered and treated, that problem needs to be accessed and attuned.

Thus, if a client experiences depression, the depressed affect has to be active to some degree at the time of diagnosis and treatment. To attune the problem, the client is simply asked to think about the problem in a way that allows her/him to get in touch with it. The presence of the energetic features of the problem, in addition to the felt emotion, can be confirmed by the client's acknowledgment and by asking the client to scale the subjective units of distress (SUD) from 0 to 10, with 0 representing an absence of distress and 10 being the highest level. Manual muscle testing can be employed in conjunction with the SUD rating, the muscle tending to weaken in response to elevated distress.[15] As a corollary, the muscle will tend to strengthen after the distress has been relieved, as well as when positive thought and emotions are attuned.

Resonance Lock

A thought field continues to resonate for a period of time after it has been attuned, even after awareness of the thought has vanished. This is consistent with our everyday experience regarding the stimulation of emotion via thought. Even after one dismisses a notably positive or negative thought that has been vividly entertained, the associated emotional response continues to reverberate for a period of time. All other things being equal, it is proposed that the length of time that the resonating continues is directly proportional to the intensity of the emotional response experienced while the thought was being consciously accessed. Thus, if the emotional intensity level of a thought is a 10 (on a 0–10 scale), it will continue to resonate twice as long as a thought that has an intensity level of 5.

However "all other things being equal" is an uncommon state of affairs. The thought field does not operate in a vacuum, immune to intervening stimuli from the client's external environment and internal experience. Therefore, one cannot be certain that the intensity and purity of the thought field will continue to resonate for a period of time sufficient to allow accurate diagnosis and thorough treatment. Allowing for this factor, my approach incorporates resonance-locking procedures, such as having the client tap on the *glabella*, as well as the *leg lock* or *pause lock* from clinical kinesiology (Beardall, 1982, 1995). These methods appear to retain "whole body informa-

---

[15] Again this applies only in the case of *double negative testing* (Diamond, 1985).

tion," so that the thought field information will entrain or resonance lock in a more enduring fashion during diagnosis and treatment (see Chapter 6).

Intentionality

Along with a number of colleagues, I have observed that one's intention has a significant bearing on the effects of tapping or touching in stimulating the energy system. Intention may be defined as the goal toward which attention is aimed or directed. The intention of the therapist and the client may serve to stimulate the energy system in positive ways. Intention is surely related to the effects of prayer, for which there is some empirical support (Dossey, 1989, 1993). Tiller (1997) has also offered some empirical support for the effects of intentionality on subtle energy. On the other hand, intentionality can have a confounding effect, in that the examiner's intention can bias the results of manual muscle testing. The therapist should therefore remain aware of this possibility in the areas of diagnosis and treatment.

Energy Balancing and More

Obviously, the essential goal of therapy is to remove the disturbance in the areas of emotions, thoughts, and behavior and to assist the individual in returning to a state of healthy psychological functioning. Here I propose that psychological disturbance can be understood in terms of an imbalance within the individual's energy system and that successful treatment is a function of restoring balance to that system. Nonetheless, even though energy is surely fundamental, it should be borne in mind that imbalance within the energy system is merely one aspect or manifestation of a psychological problem, and reinstating energetic harmony is merely one aspect of mental health. It is conceivable that one can be energetically balanced and yet behave quite badly. It is also feasible that, if other supporting systems are not adequately addressed, the effects of one's therapeutic interventions will not last.

It is tempting to adopt the theoretical position that a psychological problem is fundamentally and solely the manifestation of a disruption in the energy system that is, in turn, triggered by perturbations within the respective thought fields. Theoretically, this would mean that all that is necessary to cure the psychological problem is removal of the perturbations. That is, if the perturbations were gone, there would be nothing remaining to disrupt the energy system. There is, however, insufficient evidence to support this position and considerable clinical evidence to the contrary. Even though energetic treatments are highly effective and efficient, psychological problems treated by balancing the energy system are known to return with considerable regularity in instances of addiction, significant personality disorders, and even with some less pervasive conditions. While this can be attributed to energy toxins causing a return of the perturbations to the thought field (see chapter 12), an apparently valid consideration at times, I suspect that there are other causal factors involved. It is also insufficient to explain away therapeutic failures with circular reasoning that the perturbations must have not really been removed from the thought field or the various holons[16]; otherwise, the problem would be resolved.

Energy diagnostics recognizes the value of including cognitive and behavioral components in the overall therapeutic strategy. While it is fairly easy to alleviate psychological distress within the therapeutic encounter by instilling harmony within the bioenergy system, failure to address the patient's orientation to the future may decrease the chances of the results generalizing to needed contexts. Additionally, if you ignore the patient's level of enlightenment about the role of thought in creating experience, you miss an opportunity to assist him/her in growing in more ways than are afforded by merely removing symptoms.

With respect to generalization, this method includes what is referred to as an *outcome projection procedure*. This entails assisting the patient in orienting to specific contexts both in thought and in action, so that the results are carried over into those environments. That is, once the distress associated with the problem has been neutralized via energy balancing and removing perturbations from the thought field, the patient is asked to imagine contexts in which the symptoms tend to emerge and to project the positive results into those contexts. The patient is also trained to reapply treatment in vivo when necessary.

As an important aspect of enlightenment, the patient is educated with respect to thought awareness. While energy is fundamental, so, too, is thought. As the patient ventures into disturbing thoughts, he or she is essentially practicing unhealthy psychological functioning. Learning to recognize the connection between thoughts and feelings, as well as one's choice in such matters, is an important aspect of mental health. We assume an obligation to

---

[16] A holon is Callahan's term (borrowed from Koestler, 1967) for thought fields that comprise the psychological problem. Thus, a perturbed thought field can be made up of one or a number of holons. Each holon entails one or a number of perturbations.

educate our clients along these lines, rather than simply teaching them when and where to tap, touch, observe, etc. Also, we certainly do not want our clients to get the mistaken notion that simply stimulating energy points, as efficient as it may be at times, has greater power than they can come to realize in themselves.

   That covers some of the essential assumptions and roots of this approach. No doubt there are other assumptions operating of which I have little or no awareness at this writing. Perhaps we can assume that the best of what this method has to offer is yet to come. With this in mind, we move on to issues of preparation.

Chapter 2

CLIENT PREPARATION
AND ENGAGEMENT

And in all the seriousness of truth, hear this:
without IT man cannot live.
But he who lives with IT alone is not a man.

—*Martin Buber*

REGARDLESS OF THE APPROACH, there are a number of milieu considerations that should always be taken into account in psychotherapy. Therapy takes place in the context of a human relationship, and the characteristics and quality of that relationship are important. If the therapist proceeds on the assumption that psychotherapeutic techniques are all that matters, the quality of the relationship will suffer, as will the effectiveness of the therapy as a whole. Even when providing biofeedback, behavioral therapies, imagery exercises, energy therapies, and other approaches that rely heavily on instrumentation and/or techniques, the therapist needs to remember that the relationship is of utmost importance.

In this chapter I touch on the interpersonal features of the therapeutic interaction and cover some features specific to energy diagnostic and treatment methods. Variables such as rapport, client commitment, pacing, expectations, belief in the treatment, and the attitude of the therapist set the therapeutic stage for success or failure. The therapeutic relationship ought to be an *I-Thou*, rather an *I-It*, interaction.

19

SETTING THE STAGE FOR SUCCESS

Rapport, Empathy, and the Relationship

As early as 1913, Sigmund Freud wrote of rapport as an initial treatment goal. Regarding procedure, however, he seemed to hold that rapport would come about if the analyst had serious interest in the patient, worked on the resistances, and indicated an attitude of *"sympathetic understanding"* (Freud, 1958, p. 139).

Essentially, psychoanalytic theory considers rapport within the therapeutic context to be a transference phenomenon (Wallace, 1974). In this respect, rapport is not seen as an aspect of an authentic relationship between two individuals; but rather, the analyst is unconsciously associated with people from the past whom the client loved or admired. I am referring to positive transference here; negative transference is considered to have equivalent dynamics, minus the positive affect. Psychoanalytic theorists have investigated various factors that are conducive to the development of rapport within the therapeutic context, including the client's confidence in the therapist (Alexander & French, 1946), motivation for treatment (Dickes, 1975; Zetzel, 1956), and "basic trust" (Erikson, 1959; Wallace, 1974). Yet psychoanalysis has not provided a precise model for the development of rapport. Global concepts such as motivation, basic trust, and confidence are offered rather than exact procedures. It is assumed that the analyst will know how to create rapport if simply instructed to do so.

Besides psychoanalysts, psychotherapists in general have documented that rapport is basic to effective therapy (Bandler & Grinder, 1979; Bingham & Moore, 1959; Charny, 1966; Fiedler, 1950; MacKinnon & Michels, 1971; Menninger, 1958; O'Hanlon & Wilk, 1987; Rogers, 1942a, 1942b, 1957; Schofield, 1964; Shapiro, 1995; Sullivan, 1954; Truax, 1963). Early on both Rogers (1941) and Menninger (1958) described the therapist-client relationship as the primary goal, the essential therapeutic ingredient. Fiedler (1950) characterized effective therapy as involving an empathic, understanding environment for the client. He emphasized the importance of "the patient feel[ing] most of the time that he is really understood" (p. 241). Rogers (1957) highlighted the centrality of empathy and client acceptance to rapport enhancement and the therapeutic climate.

Considering rapport development, nonpsychoanalytic theorists have been somewhat more specific. Sullivan (1954), for instance, recommended a higher level of interaction between therapist and client than permitted by the traditional psychoanalytic posture of sitting back, taking notes, and offering intermittent interpretations. Even more specificity was evident with Rogers's method of *reflecting feelings*.

In the 1960s empirical research support for these positions emerged (Lennard & Bernstein, 1960; Truax, 1961, 1963). Truax (1961) concluded that rapport was a function of *empathy*, which he defined as "sensitivity to moment to moment feelings during the therapeutic session and the verbal facility to communicate this understanding in a language attuned to the client's current feelings" (p. 12). This definition served to highlight a heuristic set of variables. In essence, it was being suggested that rapport is a function of observable, definable language between the parties. When rapport exists, the language patterns between the communicators show certain similarities.

The similarity that Truax and others spoke of, often referred to as *convergence* or *synchrony*, was explored along a number of dimensions. Researchers noted convergence of posture (Charny, 1966; Scheflen, 1964a, 1964b, 1965), congruence of movements (Condon, 1970; Kendon, 1970a, 1970b), length of speech (Matarazzo, Weitman, Saslow, & Wiens, 1963), interruption frequency (Wiens, Saslow, & Matarazzo, 1966), pause length (Jaffe, 1967), rate of speech (Webb, 1970), and vocal intensity (Natale, 1975). These studies revealed synchrony along a number of lines when rapport is present and a dearth of synchrony when it is not.

Interestingly, these findings were transformed into techniques for creating rapport by the founders of neuro-linguistic programming (NLP). It was recommended that the therapist mirror posture and gestures and match certain verbal utterances, noting, in particular, sensory modalities (Dilts, Grinder, Bandler, DeLozier, & Cameron-Bandler, 1979). For example, it was suggested that if the client were to describe his or her experience in visual terms (e.g., "I don't have a *clear view* on what I'm aiming for in life"), the therapist might respond with visual terms as well (e.g., "I *see* that your life direction is *clearly vague* to you"). At least one study provided support for the predicate-matching strategy (Shobin, 1980). While this highly specific approach is helpful in certain respects, if taken too literally it could reduce rapport to a set of technical maneuvers.

If we turn this around somewhat, it becomes clear that the observed manifestations of rapport are not equivalent to rapport itself. Rapport comes first and is then evident in behaviors. That is, while two people in a state of rapport show certain similarities in gestures, posture, and verbalizations, it is not the same thing to say that if the therapist mimics the client's external behaviors rapport will necessarily follow. Replicating these behaviors may practically aid the therapist in entering a state of rapport, and to this extent the therapist may choose to do some "mirroring" of the client's output, but this is hardly the essence of rapport. Rather, rapport is a total state of being. When two people are in rapport, they experience a good feeling in relationship to each other. The internal sensations are positive, they experience a feeling of closeness, and their behaviors, verbal and otherwise, congruently reflect this. If a therapist wishes to enter a state of rapport with the client, all the therapist really needs to do is to appreciate the client's individuality. The therapist clears his/her mind and is open to the moment-to-moment experience of the interaction with this unique person. Negative thoughts, should they occur, are readily dismissed. In time the client and therapist come into rapport with each other.

Client Expectations and Explaining the Method

Clients enter therapy with certain expectations, another topic that has been explored in depth in the psychotherapy literature. It is generally important to elucidate the expectations early on in therapy. Is the client expecting someone else to change? Does the client expect to talk at length and in depth, using the therapist as a sounding board? Is "magic" expected? Does the client believe that the past needs to be explored in order to resolve the problem? Is the client trying to get someone off his or her back? Does the client believe that he or she can only be helped by another woman? Is a disability leave being sought? Serious strategic errors that can undermine or otherwise interfere with therapeutic progress may result from not taking the time to investigate these expectations. Elucidating these expectations can aid the therapist and client in determining what direction therapy should take, if energy therapy is appropriate, or if any therapy is appropriate at this time.

Most clients enter treatment with the desire to talk out an issue with an understanding and compassionate professional. They do not expect or desire the therapy to involve tapping on meridian points, placing their bodies in specified postures, or whirling their eyes in circles. They are not seeking energy means to therapeutic ends. Here, and elsewhere in the book, I have included statements that can be used to address expectations and inform the client about this method. One such introductory statement follows:

You've probably heard that psychological problems such as anxiety and depression are caused by stress and chemical imbalance. While not discounting the effects of the situations in your life, your relationships, and your thoughts, and acknowledging that there is certainly a chemical aspect to many problems of this nature, I can tell you that there is mounting evidence that what we call "subtle energy" also plays a fundamental role. It has been found that these energy aspects can be diagnosed by way of manual muscle checking, which involves evaluating the relative firmness in selected muscles as you touch key points on your body while bringing to mind certain thoughts and making various statements. In addition, the procedure often involves having you place one of your hands at different locations near your head, as well as turning your feet outward and moving your legs while thinking about the problem. We have found that some of the ways to successfully treat psychological problems involve having you stimulate certain acupuncture points by tapping, touching, and sometimes merely mentally focusing on them; moving your eyes in certain directions; and counting, humming, and making certain kinds of statements or affirmations. This is a partnership between us to correct energy disruptions, so that you can get relief in the areas for which you are seeking treatment. If it's okay with you, I think it would be helpful for us to evaluate and treat your particular problem in this way. Are you agreeable to such an approach?

History-Taking

Pacing is very much related to rapport and expectation. Before the therapist can forge ahead, leading the client into therapeutic territory, it is necessary to meet the client at his or her model of the world. This is not a new idea. It is an important common sense and strategic consideration. Most clients are unwilling to follow a therapist who has not taken the time to understand the essential elements of their problem. Therefore taking a clinical history not only provides relevant information for the development of a comprehensive treatment plan, but also assures the client of the therapist's professionalism and understanding of the context and origins of the problem. In short, in most instances, before the client is willing to follow therapeutic directives, he or she needs to feel understood and accepted by the therapist.

Too often, after learning a new and particularly effective technique, therapists forget about these common sense principles. Mistakenly, the technique is taken to be the "real therapy." Actually, "real therapy" includes the techniques within their context, that is, the problem and the therapeutic relationship.

Belief in the Method

It is not necessary that the client wholeheartedly believe in these treatment methods. The methodology produces results above and beyond "placebo effect." Healthy skepticism is welcome, since it helps to document the fundamental effectiveness of this approach to diagnosis and treatment. However, if the client is militantly disbelieving, this may block treatment effectiveness, and so the therapist should discuss the treatment approach in greater depth and secure permission before proceeding. Also, we must not overlook the fact that some clients simply will not accept this approach. Even if positive therapeutic results were obtained early on, some would not recognize this or would inadvertently subvert the result. Since achieving lasting therapeutic outcomes generally takes a certain amount of time, those who have a profoundly negative attitude about the method might drop out of therapy before stable results could be obtained, and then go on their way to the misfortune of themselves and others, erroneously convinced that the method has no merit. In the interest of benefiting the client, the therapist's focus ought to be on the person rather than the method. While this method is highly efficient, the therapist should possess the *requisite variety*[1] to shift in other directions to assist the client toward greater mental health. See the section below on "Skepticism and Disbelief."

Positive Expectations

While diagnosing and alleviating bioenergy imbalance appear to be independently powerful tools in the treatment of psychological disorders, there is therapeutic value in the therapist's and client's beliefs about the treatment. We might as well harness this so-called placebo effect, which essentially involves the client's innate self-healing potential. Faith in the therapeutic encounter apparently serves to increase therapeutic results, independently or in concert with the catalytic power of the energy therapy procedures (which also serve to harness the client's self-healing abilities).

Many studies have documented the effects of beliefs and expectations in a variety of contexts, while some studies have been unable to confirm these effects. The effects of experimenter expectations have been demonstrated with laboratory rats in the learning of mazes and performance in Skinner boxes (Rosenthal & Fode, 1963; Rosenthal & Lawson, 1964) and with

---

[1]This is a systems theory concept, introduced by Ashby. Van Gigch (1974) summarizes the law as follows: "The Law of Requisite Variety states that in order to control a system, a controller must be capable of taking at least as many distinct measures or countermeasures as the system he seeks to control may exhibit" (p. 377). In other words, the more choices or versatility that the therapist has available, the greater the probability that positive therapeutic results will occur.

planaria (Cordaro & Ison, 1963); teacher expectations have been shown to affect children's learning and IQ scores (Rosenthal & Jacobson, 1966); and therapist expectations have effected emotional symptom relief among outpatients (Goldstein & Shipman, 1961). Although the authors of these studies did not suggest as much, perhaps the placebo effect is really a manifestation of bioenergy being brought into harmony as a result of the profound belief that the subject and/or observer brings to the situation.

Client Commitment

In some ways the client's degree of commitment is even more important than the foregoing considerations. If one enters treatment as a result of being coerced by someone else, or even simply because he or she nonchalantly "thought it might be useful to have a consultation," little will occur in the way of therapeutic change. The client must be in the right frame of mind, one that places considerable importance on getting a personal result. In this respect it is often beneficial if the client experiences some degree of emotional distress, wanting to change certain behaviors, etc. Obviously, coming to therapy with the hope or demand that someone else do the changing is a set-up for failure. The effective therapist evaluates and instills commitment. A heart-to-heart discussion about this issue may help. Also, if the client is pathologically focused on the "need" for another person to change, taking the edge off the emotional component through energy treatments can help the individual see other creative possibilities.

Permission

The therapist should not expect a client to automatically embrace energy diagnostic and treatment methods. Permission relates to informed consent, therapeutic etiquette, and compliance; it oils the therapeutic machinery and helps to prevent resistance. And it should be borne in mind that from time to time the therapist should assess the limits of the permission given. In particular, when resistance shows up, the extent of available permission should be reviewed.

The therapist not only explains how the problem can be resolved through energy means but also secures permission to follow such a plan. If certain issues ought to be discussed, the therapist asks the client if it is permissible to "go there." Permission is often given incrementally. A court-ordered client, for example, initially may be willing only to go along with "getting to know you" and refuse to discuss the problem that initiated the referral. Next he may agree to procedures to neutralize negative emotions about being "forced" to attend sessions. Later the client may be amenable to discussions about *why* he ought to consider a behavior change and then, finally, to interventions geared to alter the behaviors themselves.

MOVING FORWARD WITH DIAGNOSIS AND TREATMENT

The Partnership

Obviously, therapy is not something done by the client or the therapist alone. It is invariably a partnership, although different approaches place more or less emphasis on one or the other partner. With this approach the therapist is the principal operator of the diagnostic procedures, although these are nonetheless conducted in partnership with the client. For example, manual muscle testing, which is discussed in detail in the next chapter, must be approached in a noncompetitive fashion if accurate information is to be obtained. After an effective means of balancing the energy system has been determined, the therapist continues to act as a guide in the session, although the client's activity becomes increasingly important. With regard to home-work assignments, such as repeating the treatments in vivo, obviously the client is primarily responsible, although the therapist remains available for input. The more cooperative the partnership, the greater the chances that significant therapeutic results will be achieved.

Attunement

In order to diagnose and treat the energetic aspects of a psychological prob-lem, it needs to be attuned. The patient is directed to "think about" or otherwise bring to mind the problem. In most instances attunement is accompanied by some degree of negative affect. This is helpful, in that it confirms that the perturbed thought field is in fact engaged and provides moment-to-moment feedback about improvements as we proceed through the diagnostic and treatment phases. Visualization is not required to attune a problem, although many patients attune most efficiently by visualizing contexts in which the problem has occurred or is prone to arise. Some patients attune via internally stored or generated auditory, visceral, kinesthetic, tactile, olfactory, or gustatory stimuli. Still others are unable to get in touch with the problem via internal cues and require specific external stimuli.

Many patients are able to access the negative emotion associated with the problem only while being in the situation where the emotion usually occurs. While there is considerable value to accessing a negative kinesthetic response associated with the problem, inability to do so does not necessarily pose a problem with regard to diagnosis and treatment. Asking the client to think about the problem in any way he or she can is often sufficient to ensure adequate attunement. In such instances the perturbed thought field can be gauged by calibrating an indicator muscle via manual muscle testing. Usually there will be a distinction between testing the muscle "in the clear" and during engagement of the thought field. The muscle response will provide the necessary distinctions to assess the specific disturbances in the energy system. After the problem has been adequately treated, the indicator muscle will test "strong" once again (i.e., as it tested "in the clear"), informing the therapist and client that the energy system is no longer in a state of imbalance in relationship to the problem.

When this approach does not prove diagnostically and therapeutically fruitful, the therapist needs to take additional measures to ensure that the perturbed thought field is adequately attuned. Often this can be achieved by assisting the client in describing the issue in considerable detail, accessing a variety of sensory modalities. We may ask the client to describe the event or recurrent problem sequentially; for example:

Therapist: (*After initially testing strong indicator muscle in the clear*) Now when you think about the accident, how do you feel on a 0–10 point scale?

Client: I really don't feel anything.

Therapist: Well, just think about it for a while. (*Therapist tests indicator muscle again and it is still strong, suggesting that problem is not adequately attuned.*) Your arm is still strong. That means we don't have this tuned in well enough yet to evaluate what is going on in the energy system. Let's try something else to see if it helps. I would like you to think about the car accident in detail now. Run it through your mind from beginning to end, paying attention to all the details you can. Try to reconstruct what you saw, heard, felt, smelled, etc. After you've done that let me know. And let me know how much distress you feel, 0 to 10, with 10 being the strongest level of discomfort.

Client: (*Runs scene through his mind for about 30 seconds*) Okay. I feel a little anxiety now. Maybe a 3 or 4.

Therapist: Now tell me about the details of the accident. And as you do, tell me what the anxiety level is from time to time. I'll ask you.

Client: I was driving along minding my own business. I came to the intersection and looked off to my left at the oncoming traffic. I saw a bus in the left-hand lane and nothing in the right lane. I turned right onto the highway and in a few seconds I heard a horn and looked at my mirror while changing gears.

Therapist: How does it feel?

Client: Stronger. About a 5.

Therapist: Okay. And then what happened?

Client: Then the windshield started cracking while the car was shaking and spinning around. I don't remember other sounds. Then the car comes to a stop and I fly out.

Therapist: How does it feel now?

Client: Stronger yet. A 7.

Therapist: We can stop there.

Client: I think I can tell you more. Might as well get it up there.

Therapist: Okay, but stop if it gets intolerable.

Client: I can see the car against a telephone pool and I'm flying through the air. I hit something and bounce. And now I'm going over a railing and hitting the sidewalk, sliding along with my feet in the air and my back against the sidewalk. Then I come to a stop and roll over. I feel that I'm bleeding inside. I remember thinking that I was going to die. It's about a 9 now.

Therapist: Now let's test your arm again. (*Therapist proceeds to test the indicator muscle, which is now relatively weak in response to this thought field. The energetic structure of the problem is now easily evaluated and effective energy-based treatments resolve the trauma.*)

Attunement vs. Exposure

It is important to distinguish between attunement and exposure. Exposure generally entails a revivification of the events or circumstances that are associated with the emotional distress. By design, exposure therapies, such as *flooding, implosive therapy,* and *emotional reliving,* produce results through abreaction and painful emoting. While such behavioral flooding has been associated with anxiety reduction (Cooper & Clum, 1989; Keane, Fairbank, Caddell, & Zimmering, 1989; Pitman et al., 1991), it has also been reported to result in undesirable side effects, such as panic, depression, and alcoholic relapse (Pitman et al., 1991).

Even though a degree of exposure may occur when the therapist directs the patient to attune a perturbed thought field, such as a painful memory, trauma, or phobia, exposure itself is not an aspect of the therapeutic process. That is, exposure is not being sought in the way that it has been utilized in abreaction therapies—to promote emotional release, desensitization, etc. Rather, with attunement the therapist's goals are to obtain a measure of the distress associated with the thought field and to lock in the thought field to facilitate energy diagnosis and treatment. Whenever possible, attunement is conducted in the absence of distressful emoting or abreaction.

If a psychological problem is to be treated effectively and efficiently, it must be attuned. Once the perturbed thought field has been attuned and locked in energetically, the patient does not need to continue consciously to attend to the psychological problem during causal diagnosis and treatment, save for intermittent reevaluations.

Measuring Treatment Effects

One efficient method to measure treatment effects is to determine subjective units of distress (SUD) on an 11-point scale. The patient attunes the psychological problem, and the therapist asks for a SUD rating. "When you think about that accident, how much does it bother you on a scale of 0 to 10, with 0 representing no discomfort and 10 indicating the highest level of distress?" This gives us a measure by which to evaluate the moment-to-moment effects of treatment. It is important that the client provide a measure of how he/she feels at the present moment, not the SUD level at the time of the trauma, usual SUD level in the real-life situation, or the SUD level the client imagines as a goal.

Some patients, particularly young children and some intellectually challenged patients, find it difficult or impossible to provide SUD ratings. Alternatively, degrees of distress can be gauged on a continuum, such as *extreme, severe, moderate, mild,* and *none.* With younger children a continuum of smiling-to-frowning faces can be used to measure degrees of distress. In other instances, the therapist may prefer simply to evaluate progress by manual muscle testing. Thus, after the muscle response has been calibrated in the clear and the perturbed thought field has been attuned, intermittent reevaluations of muscle "strength" can be used to determine when the energy system is adequately balanced. Once the thought field is no longer perturbed, muscle response should be firm.

INSURING AND EXPANDING TREATMENT SUCCESS

Skepticism and Disbelief

It is not unusual to encounter skepticism and disbelief about energy therapies. Elsewhere this has been referred to as cognitive dissonance and the *apex problem* (Callahan & Callahan, 1996; Gallo, 1998), hypothesized in terms of split-brain research and the left brain interpreter (Gazzaniga, 1967, 1985).

If the client is unprepared for energy methodology, he or she may be somewhat taken aback and accuse the therapist of "pulling my leg!" (even though most energy therapists manual muscle test on arms before ever considering legs). So, too, after the therapy has alleviated the distress of the problem, the client may conclude that this was merely an elaborate distraction, that the problem was not distressing anyway (even though it obviously was prior to treatment), or that "I'm just not able to think about it now." The highly creative client may be able to conjure up other ways to discount the results of the treatment; nonetheless, in most instances it will be clear to the client that the distress is not present, even though it may be difficult for him or her to attribute the relief to the treatment.

A little preparation can go a long way toward preventing this interference to treatment. Discussing this possibility prior to introducing the treatment is one option; however, if the therapist is congruent in providing the treatment and has good rapport with the client, even after-the-fact explanations will be acceptable to most clients. A preparatory statement such as the following may also prove helpful:

The procedure we are going to do is rather odd in many respects. One oddity is that it generally produces rapid results. Frequently, within a matter of moments one experiences significant or complete relief. This can be confusing, and some people mistakenly conclude that the distress has been relieved as a result of distraction, confusion, or something unrelated to the treatment procedure itself. I can assure you that that is not the case, and I believe you will also discover the truth of this shortly. However, if you would like, we can discuss this phenomenon in more detail later.

Challenging Results

Most therapists would not dream of asking a patient to try to become distressed once again after the distress of a trauma or some other psychological problem had been relieved. Imagine a patient who has been raped and is in treatment because of a variety of PTSD symptoms. The therapist guides the patient through a procedure, and the patient now experiences a sense of relief. Then the therapist says, "Now I want you to try your best to get upset again. Really think about it and try to recover the emotional distress you felt before." The purpose of such a directive is not to introduce a therapeutic paradox, even though in some instances that may occur. Rather, the purpose is rather straightforward: to evaluate the thoroughness of the results. If the patient is able to resurrect negative affect, the problem is not entirely resolved and additional treatment is needed. In most instances, when a patient is able to recreate the negative emotion, it will not be at the level that it was when the treatment process began. A few more efforts will usually whittle away at the remaining distress until it is gone. When the patient is able to resurrect the distress to the same level or higher than it was prior to initiating the treatment process, this is frequently due to another distinct problem or other facets of the original problem being accessed.

Layers of the Onion: Holons and Aspects

Concerning other facets, here we are often observing the proverbial layers of the onion. It is hardly news that complex psychological problems exist in various facets or layers. A recent trauma, for example, may be associated with one or a number of earlier traumas, a *trauma network*. Additionally, each trauma is generally comprised of a number of components that are interrelated with the various sub-events that took place during the summary event referred to as "the trauma" and the myriad of associated thoughts and emotions. Since there are distinctions evident at these more macro levels, there must be energetic distinctions as well. Elsewhere these distinct configurations have been referred to as *holons* (Callahan & Callahan, 1996; Koestler, 1967) and *aspects* (Craig & Fowlie, 1995a, 1995b). Even if the patient is not consciously aware of the distinctions, energy diagnosis will generally reveal the distinct structures.

Understanding that psychological disorders are ordered in this way has practical implications. Knowing that some psychological problems exist as intricate interweaves helps one to stay the course, rather than prematurely concluding that the therapy is not working. The therapist and client know that all or a majority of the aspects need to be neutralized in order to alleviate the problem.[2]

---

[2] Obviously we need to recognize when something is not working, rather than relentlessly adhering to a model that is not applicable in certain contexts. There comes a time when all models need to be reevaluated and revised as counter-examples accumulate.

Energy Toxins

In addition to related aspects or other problems, *energy toxins* can account for a resurgence of SUD. The patient is advised of this possibility and taught to track if and when the problem returns. There are various protocols used to pinpoint such toxins and to manage or neutralize them. (This is covered in detail in Chapter 12.) However, the therapist is advised not to employ the concept of energy toxins as a garbage pail explanation when therapy is not working. Other factors such as psychological reversals (Chapter 5), neurologic disorganization (Chapter 4), and negative core beliefs (Chapter 11) should be considered first.

Debriefing: Assignments, Reading, Practice, Expectations

After a problem has been effectively diagnosed and treated, debriefing is always in order. The patient needs to understand that psychological problems often need to be treated repeatedly over time and that he or she must assume an active role if lasting results are to be obtained. For many forms of psychotherapy this is not an issue, since rapid results are not experienced or expected. If the patient experiences distress (e.g., phobia, anxiety, depression, trauma, relationship problem) and in moments the distress is eliminated, the patient may become discouraged if the problem returns, unless he/she understands that this does not discount the therapy. The fact that we can eliminate the distress during the session proves that the therapy works. When the distress returns, all this means is that there is something left to treat or that the treatment did not "hold" for whatever reasons.

Besides participating in follow-up sessions specifically focused on the presenting problem, the patient is educated about the therapy as a whole and taught to repeat certain treatments if elements of the problem should arise between sessions. Specifically, the patient is taught to repeat the treatments that were effective in the office and alternatively to apply certain global treatments (see Chapter 8). It is often beneficial to recommend reading about this approach as well as to promote higher awareness of thought. In particular, I suggest books such as *Energy Psychology* (Gallo, 1998) to assist the client toward understanding energy therapies, and *Slowing Down to the Speed of Life* (Carlson & Bailey, 1998) and *The Relationship Handbook* (Pransky, 1992) to support therapeutic efforts toward instilling thought awareness.

Thought Awareness

As a fish swims through water, in all probability it has little or no conscious recognition of the water itself. It swims here and there, comes up on smaller fish or other little organisms, greets them or eats them, and goes about its business. If it should observe a bug near the surface of the water, it might swim swiftly in that direction, open its mouth wide to swallow the bug and, as it reaches the surface, fly out of the water. Momentarily the fish becomes aware of something distinct from that to which it is accustomed: the air. The contrast between air and water is enlightening. Plunging back into the water, the fish briefly realizes that it lives in water. And then once again, this awareness recedes into the background. The fish forgets.

In a sense we are similar to the fish. As we go through life there are many things of which we are unaware. Most of the time we are not consciously aware of the air, of the space between things through which we move, of the intricacies of our language, and, most of all, that we are perpetually thinking. Thought intervenes in our experience so much that it becomes our experience. All of our reality is an experience created through and of thought.

Essentially, psychological problems are manifestations of bioenergy fields and chemical, neurologic, and cognitive processes. Integral to all of this is thought. Thought occurs throughout one's body and possibly even beyond those arbitrarily defined physical limits. There are molecules of thought and emotions: neuropeptides, neurotransmitters, hormones, etc. There is specific activity occurring throughout one's brain as we think. Each thought occurs in the form of an energy or electromagnetic field, and perturbed thought fields are no different. They are merely perturbed, in that they are distinct from thought fields that are neutrally or enjoyably charged. All thought has structure and form existing at a number of levels concurrently.

While we can neutralize the charge central to a perturbed thought field by balancing subtle energies via tapping on specific acupoints, this is essentially a technique. True, it is a powerful technique, but a technique nonetheless. It is one way of balancing the energy system. While this methodology is highly efficient and effective in areas where many other approaches fail, when the therapist is treating other than delimited problems such as specific phobias and single incident traumas, he or she ought to assist the patient in also achieving a higher level of thought awareness. If the patient becomes aware that experience is a function of thought, he/she will also realize that psychological problems are also a function of thought. The patient achieves balance through the higher awareness that he/she is the generator of thought and then finds that he/she has a myriad of choices. Thus the patient learns that it is not necessary to attune perturbed thought fields related to past history, anxieties, relationship problems, etc. As the patient learns about the intricacies of his/her thinking, he/she achieves mental health.

When treating a psychological problem through energy means, the therapist, either before or after the problem has been successfully treated, discusses *thought* with the patient in ways appropriate to the individual. For example, it is often beneficial to explain that there are at least two ways to treat a trauma. One way is to remove the charge so that the memory of the event no longer has an emotional impact. Another way is to come to the realization that the trauma exists in thought and that one can choose to not generate such thoughts. In this way a healthier state of mind is maintained more steadily and in time the traumas of our lives will eventually cease to have impact. In general, it becomes easier for the patient to appreciate this after a trauma (or anxiety, depression, etc.) has been energetically treated. The patient thinks about the problem and no longer experiences distress. Now the patient is able to listen and learn. We should offer our patients the opportunity to eliminate the presenting problem and also to acquire an understanding about psychological health that can be incorporated into their everyday lives.

Chapter 3

MANUAL MUSCLE TESTING

Applied Kinesiology is based on the fact that body language never
lies. Manual muscle testing, as an indicator of body language,
enhances one's ability to observe function and its change. . . .
The opportunity to use the body as a laboratory instrument
of analysis is unparalleled in modern therapeutics,
because the response of the body is unerring.

— George J. Goodheart, Jr.

THIS CHAPTER PROVIDES details on the application of manual muscle testing
in the diagnosis and treatment of psychological problems. While manual
muscle testing can be a fairly simple and straightforward procedure, sometimes greater skill on the part of the examiner is needed. Practically anyone
can press on an extended arm or leg or attempt to separate two fingers held
together tightly. But what does one do when things do not go according to
plan? The highly skilled examiner is aware of a number of variables and is
prepared to address them when necessary. Many of those variables and
related procedures are covered here. With experience, examiners develop a
sixth sense about this process and become quicker and lighter on their feet.

MUSCLE TESTING: FROM PHYSICAL THERAPY
TO APPLIED KINESIOLOGY

Manual muscle testing originated in the field of physical therapy as a method
to evaluate nerve and muscle functions with respect to motor loss due to
conditions such as poliomyelitis and to assess the percentage of muscle
dysfunction for compensation claims. Eventually, Goodheart modified this

procedure and made it an integral aspect of applied kinesiology. In applied kinesiology, however, compared to physical therapy, muscle testing is employed in a different way and with different goals. "It is a much more discernible type of muscle testing to determine how muscle function is adapted by the nervous system" (Walther, 1988, p. 276).

Walther, a leading expert in applied kinesiology, describes the procedure as follows:

> The manual muscle test, as generally described, starts with the examiner asking the client to resist as he applies force to the patient. With the examiner's application of force, a sensation of muscle locking is perceived. With this perception, the examiner increases his testing pressure to overcome the patient's isometric contraction, taking the muscle into eccentric contraction; that is, the muscle is lengthened by the examiner's pressure while the patient continues to attempt to stop the movement. It appears that a major factor in this type of test is the ability of the patient's nervous system to lock the muscle against the examiner's pressure, and to continue adapting the muscle to meet the changing demands of the examiner's test. Often the examiner perceives a muscle as weak because it is late in adapting to his changing pressure. If the examiner applies pressure very slowly, allowing additional time for the muscle to adapt to it, the muscle will be perceived as strong. (1988, p. 277)

While a number of attempts have been made to develop instruments to objectively conduct muscle testing, thus far none has been able to duplicate the method employed by a well-trained applied kinesiologist. One of the most sophisticated muscle-testing devices, the Cybex II, measures muscle strength both isometrically and eccentrically. There are also a number of hand-held strain gauges, dynamometers, that are interposed between the examiner's hand and the muscle being tested. Some of these devices interface with computer programs to assess reliability, and others are combined with electromyography. However, it appears that what these machines measure does not correlate highly with manual muscle testing. For instance, one study found the Cybex II and manual muscle testing to be statistically independent, and another demonstrated only a .40 correlation between the two "when evaluating and correcting sacral respiratory faults" (Walther, 1988, pp. 276–277). On the basis of extensive clinical observations, it appears that the correlation between the Cybex II and manual muscle testing is strongest when the muscle weakness is the result of peripheral nerve entrapment, as compared to when the muscle weakness is secondary to causes such as a meridian imbalance.

> It appears that the major difference between testing against fixed transducers [and manual muscle testing] — whether isometric or concentric — is that the muscle is required to simply produce power [with fixed transducers]; in manual muscle testing, the muscle is required to adapt to the changing pressure of the examiner's force. This requires effective function of the gamma system adjusting the neuromuscular spindle cell, and proper interpretation of its afferent supply by the central nervous system. (Walther, 1988, p. 277)

Manual muscle testing outcomes have been shown to reflect central nervous system changes (Leisman, Shambaugh, & Ferentz, 1989). Also, significant inter-examiner reliability has been demonstrated when a single muscle is isolated for testing, but not when muscle groups are tested (Lawson & Calderon, 1997). The most sophisticated approaches to manual muscle testing have been described by Kendall and Kendall (1949), Kendall, Kendall, and Wadsworth (1971), Kendall and McCreary (1993), Thie (1973), and Walther (1981, 1988).[1] In general, these approaches are more comprehensive than what is needed when manual muscle testing is employed in the assessment of psychological problems. Less complex approaches, more suited to the purposes of the psychological examiner and psychotherapist, are described by Diamond (1980a, 1980b, 1985), Callahan (1985), Levy and Lehr (1996), and Gallo (1998).

PSYCHOLOGICALLY ORIENTED MUSCLE TESTING

Manual muscle testing in the assessment of psychological issues is rather simple and straightforward. Essentially, the examiner isolates a reasonably strong intact muscle, referred to as an *indicator muscle*, and qualitative changes in the muscle are assessed as the subject attends in consciousness to, or otherwise attunes, specific issues such as a phobia, traumatic memory, panic or thoughts of panic, feelings of depression, physical pain symptoms,

---

[1]A succinct article by Garten (1996) delineates various muscle responses observed during manual muscle testing and attempts to explain the muscle test phenomena.

and the like. Generally, when the stressful issue is attuned, a relative weakening will be discernible in the indicator muscle. Through pre- and post-test biofeedback calibration a measure of the psychological distress is obtained, as well as an analogue for evaluating therapeutic needs and treatment results. The basic therapeutic strategy involves determining what will cause the muscle to test strong. That is, which factor or factors will abolish the muscle weakness while the subject thinks of the psychologically distressing material? This assumes that there is a cybernetic relationship between the muscle response and the emotional response. Whatever cancels out the weakness may also resolve the psychological problem.

PREPARATION

In addition to general preparation issues covered in Chapter 2, specific aspects of preparation must be taken into account when conducting manual muscle testing. These are elaborated in the following sections.

Permission

It is obviously important that the therapist obtain permission from the client prior to conducting manual muscle testing and providing the therapeutic procedures that follow from such findings. Also, as an aspect of good therapeutic etiquette as well as for the sake of deterring resistance, the permission should be reevaluated intermittently. One is seldom afforded the luxury of carte blanche permission.

Since psychotherapists do not ordinarily take clients through procedures that entail some degree of touch, permission is not automatically implied by the nature of the relationship in the same way as it would be for a physical therapist, chiropractor, or medical doctor. Therefore, to provide informed consent, the therapist must explicitly convey sufficient detail regarding the procedures to the client or, in the case of a child, to his or her guardians. This requirement is distinct from standards that apply to other facets of psychotherapy which predominantly rely on verbal interactions, cognitive restructuring, guided imagery, between-session therapeutic assignments, and so on. Since such traditional mechanisms are also employed eclectically with kinesiological and energy-oriented psychotherapy, the traditional standards apply to those aspects of the treatment. While each therapist has an individual style with respect to how much explanation is offered during the therapeutic process, let me emphasize that the less universally accepted a procedure is by the field as a whole, the greater the ethical responsibility to account for one's actions.

Ethical and Legal Considerations

While the degree of physical contact during manual muscle testing is minimal — not even remotely approaching the degree of contact exercised by a massage therapist or physical therapist — it goes without saying that the psychotherapist who desires to employ manual muscle testing must be cognizant of any jurisdictional restrictions on touching a client. In time, specific ethical and legal standards will be set as increasing numbers of psychotherapists receive training and certification in this specialty area. In the meantime, it is incumbent upon the therapist who chooses to employ energy diagnostic and treatment methods to be adequately trained in the standards of such practice so as to most ethically and competently serve the client. While acquiring knowledge by reading texts of this nature is beneficial toward that end, attendance at quality seminars and workshops, in addition to extended supervision when available, is highly recommended.

Explaining the Test

So what kind of an explanation should be offered to the energy psychotherapy client? If the therapist's explanation is going to make sense, it should be consistent with the therapist's own style and with the style and educational level of the individual client. As discussed in Chapter 2, rapport is of utmost importance. Also, an explanation offered to an adult would certainly be different from one offered to an adolescent or a child. Pay attention to client questions and cues: Some clients will expect and require considerable detail; others will not be interested in much of an explanation. Nonetheless, the offer of an explanation and at least a cursory one should be provided. Some therapists may find it useful to provide the client with materials on this approach.

When working with adult and mature adolescent clients, the therapist should include the following elements in introductory statements concerning the muscle testing diagnostic method and the associated treatments:

1. Psychological problems involve many different aspects: events, situations in one's life, relationships, thoughts, beliefs, chemistry, and electrical or electromagnetic energy. The energy aspects of the gestalt may be considered to be fundamental in many respects.

2. Muscle testing (preferably referred to as *checking*, to decrease the competitive element in the client's mind) is a way of assessing the electrical or electromagnetic aspect of the psychological problem.
3. This procedure requires the therapist to minimally touch the client on the wrist and shoulder or hand, while pressing or pulling to some degree on the muscle(s) in order to assess the degree of firmness or locking in the muscle(s).
4. The client is asked to think about certain issues, events, etc., while touching various test points (i.e., alarm points) on his/her body, in order to determine what treatments are needed to alleviate the psychological problem.
5. The client may also be asked to place a hand at different locations near his/her head while a muscle is being checked.
6. The client may also be asked to place his/her feet and legs in specific positions, so as to lock certain information in the body.
7. The treatments involve the client's touching or tapping on specifically diagnosed acupoints, saying certain affirmations, and performing other maneuvers such as humming, counting, moving his/her eyes, etc.
8. Obtain the client's agreement to perform this procedure.

EXPLANATORY EXAMPLE

In Chapter 2, I offered a standard introduction for patients (p. 48). Here is an alternative, more down-to-earth explanation:

There are a lot of ideas about what causes psychological problems. Different people say that it's stress, lousy situations or events in your life, negative thoughts, or even chemical imbalance. Now, I'm sure they are all right, because all these things work together. What's more, it seems that there is also an electromagnetic part, a kind of switch that turns on the emotional problem. So if there is an awful situation in your life or if something terrible happened, you might have certain thoughts or beliefs about it, and these thoughts trigger electrical impulses in your brain and body that get the motors going that unbalance your chemistry and produce the upsetting emotions like anxiety, depression, anger, and so on. And this all feeds back into the whole shebang and keeps it going.

Now, as far as that electrical part is concerned, it seems that it can be tracked down by using a simple muscle checking procedure. You see, the muscles and nerves work together, so when you have an upsetting emotion, it causes a change in your muscles, too. The muscles tend to become firmer with positive thoughts and emotions, and somewhat looser with negative thoughts and emotions. It isn't that the muscles are really weak at such times, just that the electricity through the nerves gets interrupted so that the muscle momentarily relaxes some. The method involves checking the firmness in a shoulder muscle while you hold your arm out straight (or the muscles in your fingers as you make a circle with your index finger and thumb, etc.). I have you think about the problem you want help with to see how this affects the muscle. Then, while you continue to think about the problem, I have you touch certain places on your body, sort of circuit breakers, that tell us what to do next. This lets us know about places on your body where you need to touch or tap with your fingers to shut off the upsetting feeling. I'll also ask you to do some other things, like repeating certain phrases, moving your eyes in different directions, humming, and counting. We really need to work together cooperatively if it's going to work. Would this all be okay with you?

EXPLANATION FOR CHILDREN

Obviously, I avoid a technically involved presentation when introducing muscle testing to children. Instead, I might explain more through demonstration as follows:

Do you know about the magic arm (fingers, leg)? Come here and let me show you how it works. Is it okay for you to put your arm out like this? (The examiner demonstrates extending his/her own arm for the straight arm test. Here the examiner is also qualifying the muscle, making sure that there is no physical reason precluding this test. Alternatively, the examiner can determine which muscle to test by discussing this with the parent beforehand.) Now you do this. (The examiner gestures for the child to hold up his/her arm similarly or raises the child's arm in like manner.) While I press on your arm, you hold it up like this. (Again, the examiner instructs physically by holding the child's arm in place and pressing lightly.) See how you are able to keep your arm strong while I press on it? Now here's where the magic comes in. First I want you to say your name. Say, "My name is _____." (After the child says his/her name, the examiner presses on the arm and the arm generally remains firm.) See how your arm is still strong? Now I'd like you to pretend that you have a different name, and I'll press on your arm again. (Child says pretend name and the arm is again tested.) See how your arm didn't stay strong that time? That's the magic. Your arm always tells the truth. Now what can you think about that's really nice, like your favorite vacation or Santa Claus or something? (Child indicates preference.) Okay, good. You think about that now and I'll press on your arm again. (Arm should remain strong.) See how your arm is still strong? Now I want you to think about something else, maybe something that doesn't feel very good when you think about it. (Determine child's preference. Perhaps this pertains to the presenting problem.) Now you think about that while I check the magic arm. (Arm weakens as it is checked.) See how your arm didn't stay strong that time? Your arm only stays strong when you feel good.

The examiner can continue along these lines, checking for and demonstrating various phenomena that will be used in diagnosis. It should be noted, however, that most children under seven years of age will not be able to adapt to the requirements of manual muscle testing. In such instances, surrogate manual muscle testing is an option.

Surrogate Testing

In instances where it is inconvenient or impossible to conduct manual muscle testing directly on the client — such as with infants, young children, and seriously debilitated persons — some practitioners employ surrogate testing. This involves testing one person, the client, through another person. Although this may sound odd, if we remember the fact that electrical currents can travel through one person to another and our assumption that bioenergy exists, then it seems plausible that, if two people are in physical contact, energy and information can be linked and transferred in this manner.

Prior to conducting surrogate testing, it is important to ensure that the information being obtained is about the client and not about the surrogate. Toward this end the surrogate is first tested to determine that he/she is not neurologically disorganized and is balanced (see Chapter 4). A sample test involves challenging an intact strong indicator muscle while the potential surrogate places the *palm of one hand* atop the head.[2] After the surrogate

---

[2] This simple test quickly assesses if the person is balanced, neurologically disorganized, or massively psychologically reversed. The surrogate should not have an overenergy imbalance either. See Chapter 4 for diagnosis and correction of overenergy.

passes this test, one might test the person for his/her willingness to be a surrogate for the client. This involves having the would-be surrogate say, "I am willing to be a surrogate for (subject's name) at this time." A strong muscle response would be an affirmative. Further corroboration can be obtained by getting a "weak" response while he/she says, "I am not willing to be a surrogate for (subject's name) at this time."

Assuming that the person is a qualified surrogate, he/she remains in physical contact with the client while any of the methods described in this text are conducted. One merely treats the responses from the surrogate, assuming that they reflect information about the client.[3]

Certainly issues of rapport and permission are highly relevant with regard to surrogate testing. Additionally, such a method is so odd and voodoo-like that some detailed explanation is in order. The therapist may explain that, although this method is not widely accepted, it might be worth doing since there have been many anecdotal reports of its effectiveness.[4]

QUALIFYING THE INDICATOR MUSCLE

Essentially, qualifying the indicator muscle is a response to the question, "Is it all right for me to press on (this muscle)?" If the therapist intends to isolate the middle deltoid muscle in the shoulder region, for example, he/she will want to be certain that there is no problem with the client's shoulder, such as an injured rotator cuff. In most instances this is merely a matter of asking the client; however, one should also be alert to any difficulties that might become apparent while the test is being conducted. The client should not experience pain during muscle checking or testing. If the client were to feel pain, this would interfere with calibrating when the muscle tests "weak" as compared to "strong." Obviously, the muscle will give out easily if the client experiences pain.

---

[3] In view of the fact that the universe is literally filled with energy, it may well be that physical contact between the client and surrogate is unnecessary in order for surrogate testing to work. In this case it may be sufficient for the surrogate to simply focus his or her attention and intention on the client while the procedure is being conducted. Many practitioners have testified to the effectiveness of such an approach, for which verifying experimental studies are needed.

[4] No doubt some readers will find the notion of surrogate testing difficult or even impossible to swallow. I have experienced it to be rather disconcerting myself, even though frequently it has been accurate. When the procedure proves valid, I find myself shaking my head in disbelief. Apparently surrogate testing tweaks the boundaries of my model of reality, which in all likelihood will change in time.

Avoiding Manipulation of the Test

In preparation for conducting psychologically oriented manual muscle testing, it is of utmost importance that the examiner be in an optimal frame of mind to conduct the test. An unbiased mental set is needed to minimize the chances of unintentionally confounding the results. This optimum mind-set is referred to as the *null mental set*. Obviously, if the examiner desires specified test results, this bias will influence or force the results in the direction of the bias. The examiner also has to be careful about being overly therapeutic during the testing phase, since the subject may be so positively influenced by the therapist's demeanor as to override any possibility of accessing the problems for which he or she is seeking treatment.[5]

Although it has been proposed that the examiner's intention somehow affects the result through a resonating energy field, in most instances we do not have to look so far afield in order to recognize the quite visible mechanisms by which the intention is fulfilled.[6] For example, if the examiner believes that the subject is oriented toward unhappiness, after directing the subject to make a statement such as "I want to be happy," the examiner might be inclined to challenge the indicator muscle before the subject has completed the statement, thus catching the subject off guard and erroneously "revealing" a weak muscle response. This literal *sleight of hand*, conscious and intentional or otherwise, would then "confirm" the examiner's hypothesis. Alternatively, the unbiased examiner would be truly interested in what the muscle test had to reveal and disinterested in a preferred result. He or she would therefore properly wait until the subject had completed the statement prior to challenging the muscle.

Manual muscle testing can also be confounded as a result of the examiner's unintentionally pressing *too hard* or *too lightly*, a complaint often lodged either correctly by the astute subject or erroneously by the subject who suspects the examiner of being a fraud. There definitely are frauds in this field. I have observed some kinesiologists who demonstrate what might be called the *kinesiologist shuffle* and the *kinesiologist grunt*. These are maneu-

---

[5]If bioenergy resonates beyond one's physical body, then if the therapist is in a highly therapeutic state this will resonate to positively affect the client. It is well known among electrical engineers that if two generators are placed in proximity to each other, a regression toward the mean will occur such that the speed of slower moving generator will increase.

[6]We should not discount resonating effects of intention, which we exploit in surrogate testing. However, reason and scientific method demand parsimonious explanations.

vers whereby the examiner feigns great effort as he or she unsuccessfully "attempts" to bring down the subject's arm or other indicator muscle, appearing to come down with his entire weight after briskly skipping off the ground, this being further dramatized by a grunting sound, as if to say, "Boy, that's one strong muscle!" Of course, in such instances the examiner only appears to be exerting great effort, and if the kinesiologist is sufficiently adept at this maneuver, the subject will not be able to detect the subterfuge.

Another tactical maneuver practiced by the unethical examiner is responding in an indignant manner if the subject accuses him/her of pressing too hard or too lightly. The kinesiologist might attempt to manipulate the subject into cooperation by saying something like, "Well, if you're going to doubt my integrity, we have nothing more to do here!" The kinesiologist might also emphasize his training and experience in such matters: "I know what I'm doing here. You're mistaken!" At a more subtle level, the kinesiologist might simply laugh under his or her breath. If the subject's arm goes down too readily, the kinesiologist might again laugh and accuse the subject of not trying. Although it is not incorrect to alert the subject to "hold" the muscle firm, the manner in which the kinesiologist conveys this is all important. The goal of the unethical kinesiologist is to manipulate the subject into unquestioning acceptance of the kinesiologist's authority, hardly acceptable practice to ethical psychologists, psychotherapists, and kinesiologists.

There are times when subjects do not exert a reasonable degree of effort to maintain a firm muscle, allowing the arm to drop helplessly to the side when the phrase in question is not to their liking (e.g., "I want to have a miserable life" or "I want to remain depressed"). Of course, subjects might also recruit other muscles to lend additional support to the indicator muscle when it is "absolutely necessary" that the response be in the affirmative (e.g., "I want to have a wonderful life" or "I want to get over this depression").

To secure an accurate muscle response, it is important that the examiner and subject realize that muscle testing is a *test*, rather than a con*test*, and that consistency must be the rule. For example, if the middle deltoid is chosen as the indicator muscle, the subject's arm should be extended parallel to the floor and to the side. It should not be raised or lowered at an angle, or twisted in either direction. The hand should be relaxed, rather than in a fist. The examiner should position his/her hand at the same location on the wrist with each test. The amount of exertion time (e.g., three seconds), the speed at which the test is initiated, and the amount of pressure employed should be the same under all conditions. To alter any of these variables when testing one statement as compared to another will confound and invalidate the results.

Balancing Yourself

If the examiner is experiencing a significant degree of stress, is psychologically reversed for being able to perform the test,[7] or is neurologically disorganized[8] when he or she is attempting to do the manual muscle test, the validity of the test may be compromised. Therefore, the therapist is advised to follow the old adage of "heal thyself." Remaining in a healthy state of psychological functioning is obviously important, but even the healthiest person has off days. Being keenly aware of how one is feeling and thinking, the state of one's mood, enables one to know when it is time for a self-cleaning. The therapist might consider a global balancing procedure, such as the *over-energy correction* (see Chapter 4), in addition to maintaining "disinterest" as to the outcome of the test. The therapist can often alleviate psychological reversal for being able to muscle test a particular subject by stimulating small intestine-3 while employing the following affirmation: "*I deeply and profoundly accept myself even though I am unable to accurately muscle test.*"

Once the examiner is in balance, he or she is encouraged to trust his or her intuition and powers of observation during manual muscle testing. Often idiosyncratic phenomena come up that cannot be adequately covered here. However, any intuitions about what might be occurring with the subject during the process should be explored further with corroborative muscle testing in addition to common sense. I have made a number of discoveries in this way.

It should be remembered, however, that manual muscle testing is a test of muscle response, not a test of the *truth*. Primarily, it is a measure of the body's beliefs. It is not recommended that the examiner test something about which he/she cannot know. For example, what should we make of a positive muscle response to the statement about intelligent life existing in the star system Alpha Centauri? Or what if we were to use muscle testing as a means

---

[7]Psychological reversal, a term coined by Roger Callahan, indicates that there is a disruption in the individual's energy system that blocks the achievement of an expressed goal, such as alleviating a phobia. Similarly, an examiner can be psychologically reversed for being able to accurately muscle test. See Chapter 5.

[8]When a subject is neurologically disorganized, a disruption in communication within the nervous system exists that can interfere with, among other things, the accuracy of manual muscle testing. See Chapter 4 for detailed treatment of this topic.

of determining how many angels can dance on the head of a pin? Also, neither psychotherapists nor oncologists ought to make recommendations about cancer treatment on the basis of muscle testing results.

CONDUCTING THE TEST

A *Partnership*

One of the most important aspects of effective manual muscle testing is how the examiner-therapist frames the test. If the subject-client believes that he or she has to compete with the examiner, this will interfere with obtaining accurate information. The therapist should not simply ask the client to "resist" while the indicator muscle is being "challenged." The very fact that testing a muscle has come to be called a *challenge* has fashioned the procedure into a win-lose frame, rather than the win-win frame that it should be, especially when employed in therapy. It is not a matter of the therapist and client being in a contest with each other, the client attempting to resist the efforts of the therapist to overpower the muscle. Rather, the client and therapist should maintain a partnership. "We *together* are attempting to decipher the information stored in your body's energy system." "We *together* are trying to learn what your body knows." In the spirit of Harry Stack Sullivan, the therapist and client become *participant observers*.

With this in mind, the examiner should discuss the rationale of the muscle test, telling the client that the purpose of the test is to *discover* what is needed in order to resolve the problem for which the client is seeking consultation. Instead of using terms such as "resist" and "resistance," the examiner should request that the subject attempt to "hold" the muscle in position while it is being tested with a sufficient amount of pressure to determine if the muscle is *turned on* or *turned off*. Alternatively, the examiner might choose the words *strong* and *weak*, although the latter should be appropriately defined or intoned so as not to imply that the muscle is actually *weak*, in view of the negative connotation of weakness, which could again stir up some resistance. Again, many examiners prefer the term *muscle checking* to *muscle testing*, since the latter connotes a challenge to the subject, whereas the former does not.

Physical Positioning

If the muscle being tested is the middle deltoid of the left shoulder, the examiner stands facing the subject, lightly resting his/her right hand on

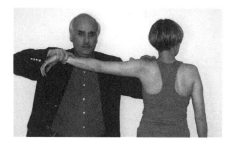

Figure 3.1 Positioning while conducting straight arm test

the subject's left wrist as the subject's arm is extended at a right angle to the left side and parallel to the floor (see Figure 3.1). The examiner stands somewhat off to the left side of the subject, avoiding close contact with subject's "energy field" at the front of the body, since this has been found to interfere with test accuracy. In some instances the examiner may choose to press his/her left hand on the subject's right shoulder in order to steady the subject (see Figure 3.2); however, this is not necessary if the examiner is able to employ sufficiently light pressure while conducting the test.

Some subjects may experience the examiner's arm across their front as uncomfortably intrusive; with them, shoulder steadying is undesirable. On the other hand, considerately asking the client if he or she would mind this approach to muscle testing is often enough to prevent discomfort that might otherwise arise. Of course, the therapist needs to be alert to clients who are overly eager to please the therapist regardless of their discomfort. In such cases it is probably best to not ask in the first place, at least not at this stage of treatment. Consider an alternative indicator muscle, such as the *latissimus dorsi* or *opponens pollicis longus*.

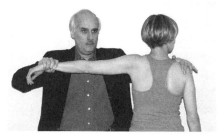

Figure 3.2 Anchoring opposite shoulder during straight arm test

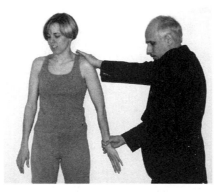

Figure 3.3 Manual muscle testing with latissimus dorsi

The latissimus dorsi may be tested by having the subject stand with an arm firm against the side with the elbow straight and the back of the hand against body. The challenge is to attempt to raise the arm away from the body (see Figure 3.3).

The opponens pollicis longus test is conducted by having the subject make an O-ring by touching the tips of the thumb and little finger to each other (see Figure 3.4). Alternatively, the thumb and index finger may be employed. The examiner attempts to pull the fingers apart. Slight separation with subsequent locking is acceptable.

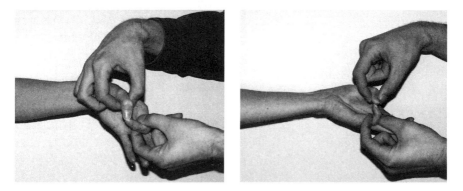

Figure 3.4 Manual muscle testing with O-ring tests

Averting Eyes

While conducting the test, it is recommended that the examiner and subject avert their eyes and do not smile or laugh, since this can interfere with the quality of the test. It stands to reason that the subject cannot effectively access the target negative state and a positive state at the same time. The positive state that is likely promoted by smiling and laughing would block attunement of the perturbed thought field.

It is generally helpful if the subject's eyes are not only averted away from the examiner but also directed down toward the floor at approximately a 45° angle. This position serves to further prevent external distractions and to facilitate the accessing of internal kinesthetics associated with the problem being treated. Meanwhile, the examiner's eyes should be averted so as to not inhibit the subject, as well as to enhance the examiner's ability to perceive felt distinctions in the indicator muscle response.

Alternatively, some prefer that both the subject and the examiner direct their gazes away from each other, to either the left or the right, while the test is in progress. This insures that neither is distracted by the other. When the subject's left arm is being tested, it is perhaps best for both subject and examiner to turn their heads and gaze in the direction to the right of the subject. In this way the subject is not distracted or inhibited by the examiner's gaze and the examiner has a good view of the subject's arm and shoulder.

Sharing Feedback

Nothing is gained if the examiner is unable to make a differentiation when testing the muscle. Generally, it is helpful for the examiner and subject to share feedback during the test. For example, when the examiner cannot determine if the muscle was stronger while the subject was touching a specific alarm point, repeating a certain phrase, or holding a substance, he/she might ask for the subject's observation. Both the subject and the examiner should be observing the muscle response to the challenge.

Sharing feedback is also an important aspect of maintaining rapport. Although I am referring to the person being tested as the "subject," this should not be construed or conveyed as a subject-object relationship. When doing effective manual muscle testing, the examiner and the "subject" are both participating observers.

Breathing

Both examiner and subject should continue to breathe normally, rather than holding their breath, during the test. If the client holds a specific phase of breathing, this may interfere with accurate assessment. For example, consider the effects of holding a phase of respiration on muscle response:

> [W]hen cranial faults are present the phase of respiration that the client takes or holds during the test has a bearing on muscle strength. In fact, individuals with disturbance in the cranial-sacral primary respiratory mechanism will innately take and hold the phase of respiration that gives optimal function to the muscle. (Walther, 1988, p. 278)

Sitting

When the subject is being tested in a sitting position, it is advisable that the subject keep his/her feet flat on the floor without crossing the legs. At times crossed legs may induce *switching* (see Chapter 4) or otherwise interfere with the muscle response. The subject should not brace by holding a hand on or beneath the chair when the opposite arm is being tested, since this action may recruit additional muscles and thus possibly impair the clarity of the test.

Calibration

Obviously it is important to be able to determine when the indicator muscle is turned on (i.e., strong) and off (i.e., weak). This is essentially an issue of calibration, of being able to make distinctions. Toward this end the subject can be asked to state his or her right name followed by a wrong name. In each instance the indicator muscle is tested. For example, if the subject's name is Jane, after the examiner has explained the purpose of the test and obtained permission to conduct it, he/she might calibrate muscle response as follows:

Examiner: I know your name, but I would like you to say, "My name is . . . " and then state your name. After you state your name, I will press on your arm and I would like you to hold it in place.

Jane: My name is Jane. (*Examiner conducts straight arm test and muscle tests strong.*)

Examiner: Good. Now I would like to check the arm after you say, "My name is Eleanor Roosevelt."

Jane: My name is Eleanor Roosevelt. (*Examiner conducts straight arm test and muscle tests weak.*)

Examiner: Did you notice those distinctions, Jane? When you said your correct name, the muscles in your arm held firm. But when you said that your name was Eleanor Roosevelt, it did not hold firm.

Jane: Yes, I did notice that. That's interesting.

A number of similar tests can be conducted to aid the therapist-examiner and client-subject in making distinctions as to muscle response. For example, the client can be asked to think about *something pleasant* and then *something unpleasant*, comparing the muscle response in each instance. Other comparison tests might include *something invigorating* (e.g., enjoying a stimulating shower) as compared to *something exhausting* (e.g., tired after a long day at work); *a truthful statement* (e.g., "I'm 46") as compared to *a false statement* (e.g., "I'm 29"), and so on. The therapist and client might also compare muscle response in relationship to antonyms to calibrate muscle response as well as the client's idiosyncratic definitions:

celebration — mourning
celebration — dishonoring
affirmative — negative
yes — no
beautiful — ugly
pleasant — unpleasant
work — play
love — hate
good — bad
happy — sad
happy — unhappy
happy — depressed
buoyancy — depression
strong — weak
relaxation — anxiety

Pressure on the Muscle

As much as possible, avoid using a lot of pressure when checking muscle response. Otherwise the chances of fatiguing the muscle increase, placing the examiner and subject at a disadvantage if a considerable amount of testing needs to be conducted. Generally, all that is needed is to determine if the muscle has locked in place. Toward this end, about two to five pounds of pressure for about two or three seconds should be sufficient. It might also be necessary to press the arm down about two inches in order to get a better sense of the muscle's capacity to hold. In most cases, pressing down any further than that is unnecessary.

Occasionally, calibration is impossible with light pressure. Alternatives include increasing pressure or even exerting enough pressure to cause a release or weakening of the indicator muscle. The examiner is advised to employ the follow-through strategy only when absolutely necessary, since this may result in discomfort and fatigue to the subject. Also, with follow-through the examiner will need to be perceptive of the differences in release response time in order to calibrate distinctions in muscle response.

Jewelry, Quartz Watches, Etc.

Sometimes the distinction between a muscle responding firm as compared to slack will be difficult if not impossible to discern due to the presence of certain kinds of jewelry, quartz watches, and other electronic devices in contact with the subject. As far as jewelry is concerned, metal necklaces and chokers, which invariably cross the midline, can result in a polarity confusion, which is also referred to as *switching*. This generally results in the muscle testing equivalently under all conditions. Metal rim eyeglasses, which also cross the midline, may interfere with test results. Simply removing the jewelry or glasses will rectify this condition. Some examiners believe that they should also remove their own jewelry to improve testing. Quartz watches, pagers, and cell phones, worn by subject or examiner, may also confuse results during muscle testing and should therefore be removed.

Hydration

If the subject is not adequately hydrated, sometimes the muscle response will not be clear, making it difficult to determine when the muscle is turned on and off. Therefore, some testers routinely have the subject drink a glass of water prior to attempting manual muscle testing. Additionally, some testers, assuming that insufficient hydration on their part can also interfere with their ability to conduct the test, routinely drink water prior to conducting the test. If the principles of surrogate testing are accurate, the contact between the examiner and subject will negatively affect the subject if the examiner is insufficiently hydrated.

The presence of subtle dehydration can be detected by a specific muscle testing procedure. If a strong indicator muscle tests "weak" while gently pulling on a small tuft of the subject's hair (e.g., at the back of the head, or an eyebrow), "dehydration" is present (see Figure 3.5). After having the subject drink a glass of water, the muscle should test strong while tugging on the hair.

Sometimes it is difficult to locate a strong indicator muscle, all the standard muscles testing weak. In this instance, after noting the weak muscle, the examiner challenges the muscle again while the subject places a couple of fingers in a bowl of water or holds some water in his/her mouth. If insufficient hydration is the cause of the weak muscle response, the muscle will now test strong. After the subject drinks some water, the muscle should now test strong while tugging on the hair. It should be emphasized that these tests do not diagnose clinical dehydration.

Deep Breathing

Sometimes having the subject take a few deep breaths will improve the quality of the muscle response, especially if the subject is considerably stressed. The breathing may help to reduce the stress and thus increase muscle strength. It should also be noted that the lung meridian is considered to be the initial or prime meridian (Diamond, 1985). Breath comes in through the lungs and stimulates energy in the lung meridian before entering the other meridians. Thus, breathing helps to increase flow of energy through the meridians, balancing the energy system and thus reducing stress.

Tapping Key Acupoints

Another way to reduce stress and thus improve muscle response is to have the subject tap on a few acupoints relevant to the source of the stress. Tapping

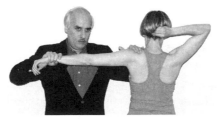

Figure 3.5 Kinesiologic hydration test

directly under the eyes (stomach-1), four inches under the armpits (spleen-21), and under the collarbones next to the chest bone (kidney-27) can often help to reduce generalized stress. Tapping on the inside tip of a little fingernail (heart-9) may help to reduce stress related to anger. Tapping or rubbing at the beginning of the eyebrows near the bridge of the nose (bladder-2) may help to reduce feelings of frustration, impatience, or restlessness (Gallo, 1998).

Signaling When Ready

Some clients are consistently caught off guard when we challenge the indicator muscle. In such instances, it is useful for the subject to alert the examiner when he or she is ready to be tested. For example, the subject can say "ready," "push," or "okay" when he/she is ready for the examiner to push on the muscle.

Elucidation of the Subject's Thoughts and Feelings

At times, difficulty conducting the test is due to what the subject thinks and feels about the procedure. In this regard it can be useful to ask the subject if he/she has any idea what might be interfering. For example, "Usually this works pretty well. Do you have any idea what might be going on?" A little discussion can often go a long way toward resolving the subject's concerns and/or assisting the therapist in making needed adjustments.

Strategies When Muscles Invariably Test Strong or Weak

If the subject's muscle response is invariably weak, sometimes simply asking the subject to hold the muscle firmer will rectify the problem. Likewise, if the muscle response is invariably strong, so that a distinction cannot be made, asking the subject to employ less "resistance" will make for more informative muscle testing. In this respect, it is often helpful to ask the subject to give a third of his/her strength.

Located in the belly of each muscle are *spindle cells*, which monitor muscular contraction and extension. If the muscle is overcontracted, the spindle cells send a signal to the central nervous system to "switch off" the muscle, thus resulting in a releasing of the constriction. This natural mechanism can be manipulated by the examiner to improve the quality of manual muscle testing. Thus, if the muscle invariably tests strong, the examiner can turn off the muscle by pushing the belly of the muscle together a few times, thereupon causing the muscle to test weak. On the other hand, if the muscle chronically tests weak, the examiner can turn on the muscle by pressing at its center and separating in the direction of the opposite ends, toward the origin and insertion.[9] By demonstrating the distinction of strong and weak responses to the subject in this way, more accurate muscle responding can be obtained. In addition, an overly constricted or overly extended muscle can be corrected. (See Figure 3.6.)

Another way to adjust a muscle that tests consistently "weak" or "mushy" is by having the subject hold one hand over the *anterior fontanel* (i.e., the location of the soft spot on the heads of infants) while rubbing the neurolymphatic reflexes between the second and third ribs adjacent to the sternum or breast bone (see Figure 3.7). This is done for approximately 20–30 seconds, after which muscular response is again assessed. Frequently this will result in the muscle responding in a firmer manner.

Often a muscle that tests consistently "weak" or "mushy" can also be corrected by having the patient tap in a horizontal oval shape above either ear along the *temporal sphenoidal (TS) line* for approximately 10–20 seconds (see Figure 3.8). M. L. Rees defined the TS line, and Goodheart later associated various points along it with organs, glands, and muscles (Walther, 1988). After conducting the *temporal tap*, the muscle response will frequently become firmer.

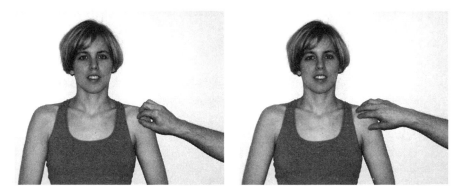

Figure 3.6   Spindle cell maneuver

---

[9]The *origin* of a muscle is the end where there is a more fixed attachment, whereas, the *insertion* is the end attached to the bone that it moves.

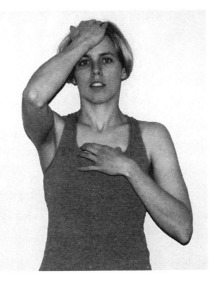

Figure 3.7 Correcting for weak muscles via anterior fontanel

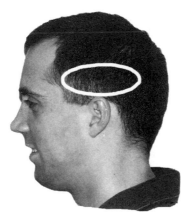

Figure 3.8 Temporal sphenoidal line

Neurologic Disorganization/Switching

If the indicator muscle consistently tests strong, with no observable distinction between positive and negative statements, pleasurable and painful thoughts, valid and invalid reports, etc., neurologic disorganization, also called switching, may be present. When this condition exists, the indicator muscle will not respond to treatments directed at spindle cells and other approaches described in the present chapter. As long as switching is present, accurate manual muscle testing is obviously impossible, since distinctions in muscle response cannot be made. Therefore, switching must be at least temporarily alleviated if we are to proceed to use this tool in the client's service. Chapter 4 presents detailed diagnostic and treatment methods specific to this phenomenon.

Chapter 4

BLOCKS TO TREATMENT EFFECTIVENESS I: NEUROLOGIC DISORGANIZATION/SWITCHING

> The nerve cells in the human brain are sufficiently sensitive
> to register the absorption of a single photon.
>
> — *Danah Zohar*

THE PHENOMENON of *neurologic disorganization*, also referred to as *polarity switching* or simply *switching*, is a significant block to energy diagnostic and treatment effectiveness. This condition is singularly relevant, since, in addition to impeding therapeutic progress, it is often consistent with physical awkwardness, difficulties with coordination, problems with directionality, and learning difficulties. Neurologic disorganization makes it impossible to accurately calibrate muscle response, to determine when a muscle response is "strong" or "turned on" and when it is "weak" or "turned off." Therefore, manual muscle testing diagnostics, other than the specific procedures used to assess neurologic disorganization itself, cannot be accurately conducted until this condition is at least temporarily moved to the side, corrected long enough so that the examiner can proceed.

> When using manual muscle testing as an indicator for therapeutic approach, it is necessary that the nervous system be organized to provide correct information; otherwise, therapy might be directed to the wrong area. Disorganization may also result in failure to find dysfunction, or may indicate problems that are not actually present. (Walther, 1988, p. 148)

The information contained in this chapter, besides having relevance to overall physical and psychological functioning, is also crucial to the effective use of the diagnostic and treatment protocols that follow.

MUSCLES AND NEUROLOGIC DISORGANIZATION

The functioning of muscles in healthy, neurologically organized people shows consistently predictable characteristics. Most muscles are paired, so that one side tenses or facilitates when the opposite side relaxes or inhibits. Thus, alternating facilitation and inhibition of the sternocleidomastoid, neck flexors (i.e., anterior scalenus, middle scalenus, posterior scalenus, longus capitis, and longus colli) and neck extensors (i.e., splenius capitis and cervicis, semispinalis capitis and cervicis) make it possible for us to move our heads in various directions. This process is also apparent with more complex movements involving groupings of muscles, such as walking, running, dancing, or swimming. Various muscles alternatively strengthen and weaken in order to make smooth, ongoing movement possible.

The coordinated action of muscles is mediated by the spinal cord and the central nervous system through an intricate interplay of afferent[1] and efferent[2] signals. The various sensory receptors send signals to the central nervous system, which in turn regulates facilitation and inhibition of the respective muscles in a coordinated, organized fashion. When conflicting afferent signals are sent to the central nervous system — as a result of structural, chemical, or mental factors — the person becomes neurologically disorganized. Here is an example of how structural imbalance can produce neurologic disorganization: If pencils are positioned beneath the great and little toes of one foot, in the direction of the heel, subluxations will be simulated, thus disrupting normal afferent signals to the central nervous system (see Figure 4.1). Running a manual muscle test of neurologic disorganization under such conditions will often yield positive results. (See various diagnostic tests outlined below.)

When the muscles function in a disorganized fashion, this is often an indication of neurologic disorganization. It appears to entail disorganization of the cerebral hemispheres, as well as bodily polarity imbalances. Disorgani-

---

[1] Afferent or sensory neurons conduct impulses from the periphery of the body to the brain or spinal cord.

[2] Efferent or motor neurons conduct impulses from the central nervous system or spinal cord to effectors, either muscles or glands that are capable of responding to the nerve impulse.

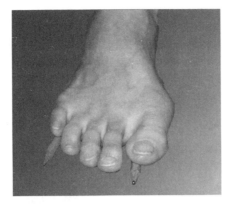

Figure 4.1   Pencils under 1st and 5th metatarsals to simulate switching

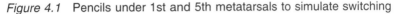

zation between the hemispheres and the body's bilateral symmetry is consistent with right side/left side polarity imbalance. Polarity imbalance can also occur with respect to anterior/posterior (i.e., front/back) and the superior/inferior (i.e., top/bottom) directionality. These polarities obviously correlate with the three dimensions of length, width, and height.

CLINICAL SIGNS OF NEUROLOGIC DISORGANIZATION

Clinical signs indicative of neurologic disorganization include reversal of letters and numbers, confusing left and right, saying the opposite of what one means, various difficulties with spatial directions, and so forth. Switching is relevant to learning problems and is also similar in some ways to *psychological reversal* (see Chapter 5).

Significant physical awkwardness or clumsiness can also be a sign of neurologic disorganization. Noticeably, the neurologically disorganized person may show increasingly curtailed arm movement or even an absence of arm swing altogether when walking; in the most extreme cases ambulating will be characterized by homolateral coordination of arms and legs, most typically present when running, rather than the normal heterolateral movement.

When the client is switched, psychological problems are generally slow to respond and even recalcitrant to energy-based treatments and perhaps therapies in general. Therefore correction is required to facilitate treatment.[3]

---

[3] There are some anecdotal reports that correcting neurologic disorganization with methods described in this chapter also facilitates cognitive retraining.

CAUSES OF NEUROLOGIC DISORGANIZATION

One of the primary causes of switching is cranial movement dysfunction. When impaired movement among various cranial bones, which also affects respiration and flow of cerebrospinal fluid, is the cause of switching, it must be corrected; otherwise, the dysfunction will remain.[4] One approach to treating switching involves *cranial-sacral therapy*, a rather complex procedure employed by some osteopathic and chiropractic physicians that in part focuses on alleviation of cranial faults. This therapy also addresses movements that occur in the vicinity of the pelvis and sacrum during respiration.

Other causes of switching include chemical toxins, severe psychosocial stress, and structural imbalance caused by such anomalies as fallen arches, improperly fitted lower extremity prostheses, and various subluxations. Each of these must be thoroughly addressed if switching is to be ameliorated. A basic principle of applied kinesiology and other holistic approaches is that dysfunction can result from any one or combination of factors from the structural-chemical-mental *triad of health* (Palmer, 1910).

While the methods described in this chapter are highly useful in diagnosing neurologic disorganization and temporarily (and sometimes substantially) correcting it, generally this condition cannot be corrected in any permanent way through these methods, especially when an energy toxin, nutritional deficiency, or structural imbalance is responsible for the neurologic disorganization. In such instances correcting the primary cause will simultaneously reestablish neurologic organization. (See Chapter 12 for methods of diagnosing and treating exogenous toxins.)

DIAGNOSING NEUROLOGIC DISORGANIZATION

In addition to observing the clinical signs of neurologic disorganization, one can conduct various fairly simple manual muscle tests to verify its presence. We must be able to determine when a patient is switched so that this condition can be at least temporarily ameliorated, since correction makes it possible to effectively conduct other relevant diagnostic and treatment methods. What follows is a number of the most relevant tests of neuro-

---

[4] There are 14 potential cranial faults, any of which can misalign and impair functioning in various ways, including causing neurologic disorganization. The cranial bones move with breathing, as does the sacrum.

logic disorganization/switching, arranged from the most basic to the most complex.

True-False Method

A basic screening test of neurologic disorganization occurs when the indicator muscle tests equally firm after the client makes a true statement as compared to a false statement, such as stating his or her correct name and then an incorrect name, for example, "My name is Fred Gallo" followed by "My name is Benjamin Franklin." Other true-false statements can also be used (e.g., what the subject ate for breakfast, the subject's age, height, weight, birth place). Normally, one would expect the muscle to respond with firmness to the true statement and relative weakness to the false one. When the muscle response is equally firm under both conditions, which means that neither the examiner nor the subject can observe a response distinction, the possibility of switching exists. Since an equally strong muscle response can be due to other factors, such as the client being highly adept at telling lies, the examiner should follow up this screening test with a more sophisticated test of neurologic disorganization.[5]

Hand-over-Head Method

A somewhat more advanced means of screening for neurologic disorganization, the *hand-over-head* screening test is conducted by having the client place the palm of his or her right hand about an inch above the apex of the head while the examiner tests the strength in the extended left arm (middle deltoid group) or any other indicator muscle. If distinctions between muscle responses are not otherwise evident, this screening test will generally not provide any additional useful information; however, when there is a subtle difference between "strong" and "weak" muscle responses, such that the examiner finds it a difficult if not impossible call, this test can often clarify the results. If the client's indicator muscle tests strong when the palm

---

[5] Statistics on the accuracy of polygraphs range from 80%–98%, depending upon the studies reviewed. Inaccuracies may be due to errors in interpretation, preparation of subjects, and other confounding variables. While there are also inconclusive results with polygraphs that should not be considered instances of inaccuracy, some reviewers have included such statistics, thereby lowering the accuracy ratings. While manual muscle testing is a more complex procedure than a polygraph, these same considerations apply.

is positioned over the head and weak when the back of the hand is positioned over the head, neurologic disorganization is precluded in most instances. If there is no distinction between the *palm down* and *palm up* positions, neurologic disorganization is a distinct possibility. If the palm tests weak and the back side tests strong, this may be an instance of so-called massive psychological reversal (see Chapter 5 for details). A useful mnemonic device for determining that the client is not neurologically disorganized is described by Durlacher (1994): "palm is power; back is slack."

The distinction between *false negative* and *false positive* is relevant here. In the case of a false negative, the test results indicate that the phenomenon under scrutiny is *not present* when in fact it is. In the case of a false positive, the test indicates that a disturbance *is present* when in fact it is not. In the author's experience, the hand-over-head screening test seldom produces false negatives, although some false positives can be expected. Therefore when this test suggests the presence of neurologic disorganization, it should be followed up with a more sensitive test (see below).

As noted, the body appears to be variably polarized head to foot, side to side, and front to back. If one is normally organized, the back of the hand is positively charged and the palm is negatively charged, while the head is positively charged and the charge at the feet is negative. Thus the charge is uninterrupted with the individual who is neurologically organized when the palm is placed atop the head, a "strong" muscle response being evident. If the polarity on the hand is reversed, but not so on the head (or vice versa), a competing electromagnetic situation will exist, similar to when like magnetic poles are placed in contact with each other. Since this situation interferes with the normal electromagnetic flow, we observe opposite effects. In order for the indicator muscle to remain strong under both conditions, it would seem that either or both of the hand and head polarities must be neutralized.

Index Finger Method

A third, somewhat more comfortable diagnostic test, based on the same principles and considerations as the hand-over-head method, involves either the client or tester placing the palm side of an index finger at the bridge of the client's nose while testing the arm. The indicator muscle should test strong under this condition. On the other hand (or finger, if you will), when the nail side of the finger is placed at the bridge of the nose, the indicator muscle should test weak. If the indicator muscle remains strong under both conditions, neurologic disorganization is possibly present. If the palm side tests weak and the nail side tests strong, similar to the hand-over-head method, this may also be indicative of massive psychological reversal (see Chapter 5).

Ocular Lock

Many therapists who practice thought field therapy (Callahan, 1985), eye movement technology (Johnson, 1994), eye movement integration (Andreas & Andreas, 1995), and eye movement desensitization and reprocessing (Shapiro, 1995) have no doubt observed the phenomenon referred to as *ocular lock*, a disturbed coordination of the eyes. This can be seen when the patient is directed to rotate his/her eyes 360°, tracking the examiner's finger or a hand-held object. If a jerky, saccadic eye movement is observed at one or several points along the rotation, ocular lock and neurologic disorganization may be indicated. When the eyes are held at the precise location of the saccadic movement, given ocular lock, a previously strong indicator muscle will weaken. In such instances the indicator muscle will also weaken while the patient's eyes follow the therapist's finger in either or both clockwise and counterclockwise 360° directions. In instances of ocular lock, frequently the indicator muscle will also weaken while therapy localizing to K-27. According to Walther (1988), ocular lock is usually evidence of a cranial fault.

Some of the indicators of ocular lock and neurologic disorganization are:

1. A lack of coordination of the eyes is evident; however, this may be related to factors other than ocular lock (e.g., strabismus caused by eye muscle weakness).
2. A strong indicator muscle weakens after or while the eyes are being rotated 360° in either or both clockwise and counterclockwise directions. Muscle weakening usually occurs in one direction, although it occasionally occurs in both.
3. When ocular lock is present, often there will be indicator muscle weakening while therapy localizing K-27.
4. While the subject's eyes track the examiner's finger 360° in either clockwise or counterclockwise directions, saccadic eye movements will be observed at a specific location along the rotation.
5. When the subject's eyes are held at the location of the saccadic movements, a strong indicator muscle will weaken.
6. Since ocular lock is usually caused by a cranial fault, cranial manipula-

tion may be required in order to rectify the condition. However, generally the ocular lock and neurologic disorganization can be at least temporarily corrected by methods such as *K-27-umbilicus, conception vessel-governing vessel*, and the *collarbone breathing exercises* discussed later in this chapter.

K-27 Therapy Localization Method

A fifth test of neurologic disorganization involves either the therapist or client therapy localizing to the K-27s. This is done by placing the tip of either index finger (or index and middle fingers) directly beneath a clavicle at a K-27 point, also referred to as the *collarbone point* or cb, while testing the indicator muscle (see Figure 4.2). These points are located immediately next to the sternum and at the juncture of either clavicle and first rib. Neurologic disorganization is probably not present if the indicator muscle remains strong while therapy localizing K-27. If the muscle weakens, neurologic disorganization may be present. The tester should bear in mind that positive therapy localization in the vicinity of K-27 can also be due to conditions other than neurologic disorganization, such as an active neurolymphatic reflex in the K-27 vicinity or a subluxation of the first rib or of the sterno-clavicular articulation (Walther, 1988); therefore, care should be taken to ensure that the patient is touching precisely at the K-27 point.

One should test both K-27 points. If either point causes the indicator muscle to test weak, switching is possibly present. Repeating this test after providing one of the neurologic disorganization corrections discussed below will result in the muscle testing strong, assuming that the condition has been successfully alleviated.

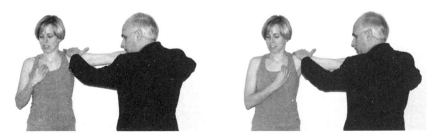

Figure 4.2   K-27 therapy localization

K-27 Therapy Localization with Phases of Breathing

An even more precise method of diagnosing neurologic disorganization involves therapy localizing each of the K-27 points with both sides of each hand in conjunction with five distinct phases of breathing:

1. normal respiration
2. deep inspiration
3. half expiration
4. deep expiration
5. half inspiration

Therapy localizing and challenging K-27/breathing in this manner is an advancement over simply therapy localizing K-27, since it takes into account the fact that neurologic disorganization is often related to cranial faults, which are also interrelated with respiration. This method is even further advanced by taking into account front-back and right-left polarity distinctions, therapy localizing each of the K-27 points with both sides of the hands. Specifically, each phase of breathing is challenged under each of the following conditions:

1. palmer side of left index finger tip at left K-27
2. palmer side of left index finger tip at right K-27
3. palmer side of right index finger tip at left K-27
4. palmer side of right index finger tip at left K-27
5. knuckle of left index finger at left K-27
6. knuckle of left index finger at right K-27
7. knuckle of right index finger at left K-27
8. knuckle of right index finger at right K-27

Therapy localization with phases of breathing and left-right and front-back polarities discloses some of the elements relevant to "hidden switching" (i.e., switching that does not manifest until a specific activity or condition is present). After diagnosing in this manner, the therapist can provide one of the methods described below to at least temporarily alleviate the neurologic disorganization. However, it is most efficient and often necessary to direct the treatment to one of the 40 diagnostic elements (i e., five phases of breathing multiplied by eight finger/K-27 positions). One way to fulfill this requirement is to provide the *collarbone breathing exercises* (Callahan, 1990), described below, in conjunction with manual muscle testing diagnosis.

CORRECTING NEUROLOGIC DISORGANIZATION

A number of methods to correct neurologic disorganization and thereby facilitate manual muscle testing and enhance therapeutic results are described below. These methods do not necessarily address the fundamental cause of the problem, which may be related to structural, chemical, and mental factors. To thoroughly alleviate neurologic disorganization, therapy specifically directed at the cause is often needed.[6] Nonetheless, these methods are relevant for the applied kinesiologist as well as the psychotherapist.

Patterned Walking

When the client diagnosed with neurologic disorganization also shows curtailed or absent heterolateral arm swing while walking, sometimes the disorganization can be temporarily alleviated by having the client consciously practice walking with heterolateral arm swing for a few minutes. The therapist should model and coach the client through this procedure, since it is generally difficult, if not impossible, for clients with the most extreme form of this condition to practice the pattern simply through verbal instruction. Once the client has had sufficient practice with the therapist's assistance, it is often beneficial to assign this exercise on an ongoing basis between sessions.

K-27-Umbilicus Protocol

While exploring the interrelationship of specific muscles and acupuncture meridians, Goodheart discovered that neurologic disorganization could be at least temporarily corrected by stimulating the last point on the kidney meridian (KI-27 or K-27) along with the umbilicus (Walther, 1988) (see Figure 4.3). When manual muscle testing results are unpredictable and there are other indications of neurologic disorganization, such as positive therapy localization to K-27 and positive ocular lock, simultaneously stimulating the K-27 points and the umbilicus will often result in a correction that will hold sufficiently for diagnostic and some treatment purposes. While

---

[6]Sometimes these methods do substantially correct neurologic disorganization in an ongoing way, even though the fundamental cause of the disorganization has not been thoroughly diagnosed. In such cases the correction essentially occurs by accident rather than by design, since the treatment was not specifically and precisely directed at the underlying cause.

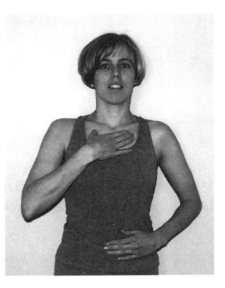

Figure 4.3   K-27 umbilicus protocol

more detailed methods based on this finding are presented later, the basic K-27-umbilicus protocol follows:

1. Results of manual muscle testing are inconsistent and a strong indicator muscle weakens while therapy localizes either K-27 point. There may also be a positive ocular lock, detectable by having the client rotate the eyes 360° while following the examiner's finger. Ocular lock is evident by a saccadic movement of the eyes at some point(s) along the rotation. (See diagnostic procedure described above.)
2. Have the client vigorously tap or rub each K-27 point in turn for about 20 seconds, while also vigorously stimulating or simply placing the free hand over the navel.
3. If K-27-umbilicus has corrected for neurologic disorganization, manual muscle testing results will now be predictable.
4. Also, if this has corrected for neurologic disorganization, a strong indicator muscle will remain strong while therapy localizing the K-27 points (i.e., negative therapy localization).
5. If treatment has been effective, any positive ocular lock that was found prior to the treatment will now be eliminated. The indicator muscle will now remain strong while challenging the eye position that previously resulted in a weakening of the indicator muscle.

Auxiliary K-27-Umbilicus Protocol

Contiguous and bilateral to the *transverse processes* of 11th thoracic vertebra (T11) are the auxiliary K-27 points.[7] These points can be used as alternatives to the K-27 points for diagnosing and treating neurologic disorganization (see Figure 4.4).

1. Results of manual muscle testing are inconsistent, and a strong indicator muscle weakens while therapy localizes either auxiliary K-27 point. There may also be a positive ocular lock, detectable by having the client's eyes track the examiner's finger 360°. Ocular lock is evident when a saccadic movement of the eyes occurs at some point(s) along the rotation. (See diagnostic procedure for ocular lock described above.)
2. Vigorously tap or rub each auxiliary K-27 point in turn for about 20 seconds each, while also stimulating the umbilicus.

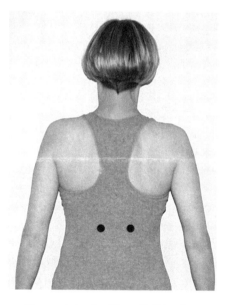

Figure 4.4   Auxiliary K-27 points

---

[7]There are 12 thoracic vertebrae, preceded and followed respectively by seven cervical and five lumbar vertebrae. These are followed by five sacral and four coccygeal vertebrae. The transverse processes are the bony extensions of the vertebrae that extend crosswise.

3. If auxiliary K-27-umbilicus has corrected for neurologic disorganization, manual muscle testing results will now be predictable.
4. If the treatment has corrected neurologic disorganization, a strong indicator muscle will remain strong while therapy localizing the auxiliary K-27 points (i.e., negative therapy localization).
5. If treatment has been effective, any positive ocular lock that was found prior to the treatment will now be eliminated. The indicator muscle will now remain strong while challenging the eye position that previously resulted in a weakening of the indicator muscle.

Nasal Tap

Frequently neurologic disorganization can be temporarily corrected by having the patient tap rapidly for approximately a minute simultaneously on both sides of the bridge of the nose (see Figure 4.5). The *nasal tap* often corrects for switching long enough so that diagnosis and treatment can effectively follow. In view of the fact that it has been proposed that neurologic disorganization is often related to cranial faults, perhaps this method works by making a correction in this area (Walther, 1988).

The nasal tap can be used as a further test and correction for neurologic disorganization after a positive ocular lock has been found and either the K-27-umbilicus or auxiliary K-27-umbilicus treatment has been provided. The protocol proceeds as follows:

1. Locate a positive ocular lock as described above.
2. Treat the ocular lock/neurologic disorganization with the K-27-umbilicus method.

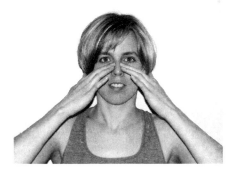

Figure 4.5 Nasal tap

3. Test an indicator muscle after having the patient take two quick nasal sniffs while positioning the eyes in the direction where the positive ocular lock was found.

4. If the indicator muscle weakens, have the patient tap rapidly for approximately a minute on both sides of the bridge of the nose.

5. After treating with the nasal tap, the indicator muscle should remain strong after the patient takes two quick nasal sniffs while positioning the eyes in the direction where the positive ocular lock was previously found.

Three Polarities Unswitching Procedure[8]

Switching/neural disorganization appears to involve body polarities. Think of this as a direct current that travels from positive to negative poles. In this respect there are three areas in which polarity can be switched: left-to-right polarity, front-to-back polarity, and top-to-bottom polarity. The following procedure, illustrated in Figure 4.6, specifically addresses all three of these aspects of polarity:

1. Have the client stimulate the umbilicus by pressing on it with the first three fingers of either hand while briskly tapping or rubbing with the fingers of the free hand under both collarbones next to the sternum for about ten seconds (Figure 4.6a).

2. Next have the client continue to stimulate the navel while tapping or rubbing under the nose for about ten seconds (Figure 4.6b).

3. Next have the client stimulate the umbilicus while tapping or rubbing under the bottom lip for about ten seconds (Figure 4.6c).

4. Finally have the client stimulate the umbilicus while rubbing the coccyx for about ten seconds (Figure 4.6d).

5. Reevaluate for switching.

Over-energy Correction

Neurologic disorganization can result from over-energy in the meridians. When the central vessel, one of the two midline meridians, is overenergized, the individual may report feeling "confused," "spaced out," or unable to

---

[8]The three polarities unswitching procedure was called the basic unswitching procedure in *Energy Psychology: Explorations at the Interface of Energy, Cognition, Behavior, and Health* (Gallo, 1998).

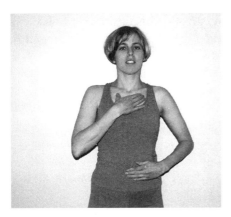

(a)

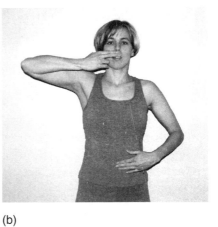

(b)

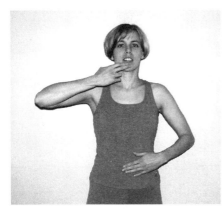

(c)

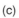

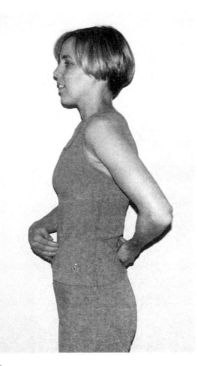

(d)

Figure 4.6 (a–d)   Three polarities unswitching procedure

concentrate. The presence of over-energy can often be diagnosed by locating a strong indicator muscle, having the client quickly trace the central meridian upward from the pubic bone to the chin three times with the palm of a hand and then rechecking the indicator muscle, which should test strong. Opposite results indicate over-energy. Next, tracing the meridian downward three times should result in the indicator muscle testing weak. Opposite results are indicative of over-energy. No distinction between the muscle tests is also suggestive of neurologic disorganization and possibly of over-energy.

One method of correcting for over-energy and associated neurologic disorganization is by having the client perform the following exercise, illustrated in Figure 4.7:

1.   Interlock ankles, placing left ankle over right.
2.   Place hands out in front, arms extended, with backs of hands touching.
3.   Bring right hand over left hand and then hold palms together.
4.   Clasp/enfold fingers.
5.   Fold hands and arms inward and rest on chest, underneath chin.
6.   Breathe deeply while resting tongue against upper palate behind center ridge.
7.   Reevaluate for switching and over-energy after one to two minutes of this exercise.

Connecting Conception Vessel–Governing Vessel

Another method of correcting for energy disruptions related to or causative of neurologic disorganization is by balancing the energy movement between both midline meridians, the central vessel (CV) and the governing vessel (GV) (see Figure 4.8). Neurologic disorganization related to these meridians can be diagnosed by indicator muscle testing while therapy localizing GV-26 and then CV-24. The client places the palm side of an index finger under the nose (GV-26) while a strong indicator muscle is tested, a weak response indicating that there is a disruption in that vessel. The energy pattern in the central vessel is similarly assessed by having the client place the palm side of an index finger directly under the bottom lip (CV-24). When there is positive therapy localization to either of these points, correction can be made by having the client follow these steps:

1.   The client simultaneously presses on CV-24 (under bottom lip) and CV-2 (upper symphysis pubis) for approximately 30 seconds, followed by 30 seconds of pressure simultaneously on CV-2 and GV-1 (tip of the tailbone or coccyx).

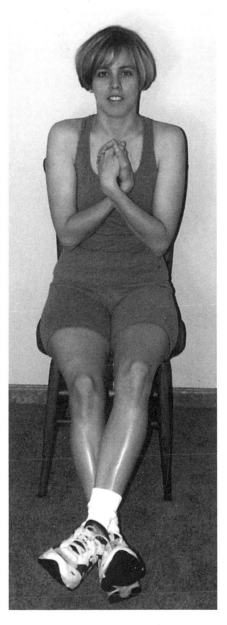

Figure 4.7 Over-energy correction

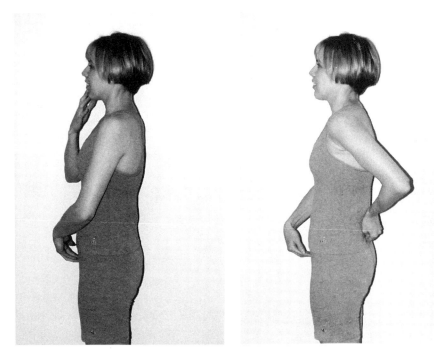

Figure 4.8   Connecting conception vessel and governing vessel

2. If this procedure results in a correction of neurologic disorganization, therapy localization to CV-24 and GV-27 will be negative and manual muscle testing will now be predictable.
3. If this procedure is effective, therapy localization to K-27 will be negative and ocular lock will also be alleviated.

The Collarbone (K-27) Breathing Exercises

Developed by Callahan (1990), the *collarbone breathing exercises* (CBB)[9] provide another way to rectify neurologic disorganization. Clients evidencing rather recalcitrant neurologic disorganization may be prescribed this proce-

---

[9]The *collarbone breathing exercises* are more accurately referred to as the *K-27 breathing exercises*, since it is the K-27 point and not the collarbone or clavicle itself that is therapy localized during treatment. The treatments will not be effective unless they are directed to the K-27 points.

dure on a regular basis, independently of or preceding other treatments specifically directed at the presenting psychological problem.

This treatment approach involves simultaneous stimulation of the *triple energizer meridian* at TE-3[10] (located between the little finger and ring finger metacarpals on the back of the hand), and the *kidney meridian* at K-27[11] (located under the clavicle or collarbone on either side of the sternum or chest bone) while directing the client through a fairly elaborate breathing routine. The entire procedure can be provided in a shotgun fashion (see Gallo, 1998), although more precise attention to the individual components is often needed in difficult cases. When these exercises are provided in conjunction with diagnosis, K-27 therapy localization with phases of breathing, as described earlier, is employed.

When conducting the exercises without precisely directed diagnosis, the subject begins by placing the palm side of the *tips of the left index* under the *left* K-27 next to the sternum while steadily tapping on TE-3 of the left hand with the index and middle finger tips of the right hand. During the tapping procedure the subject engages in five distinct breathing positions, simultaneously tapping five to seven times during each of the following phases of breathing:

1. normal respiration
2. deep inspiration
3. half expiration
4. deep expiration
5. half inspiration

After completing this phase of the treatment, the same tapping and breathing procedure is repeated while having the client place the palm side of the *tip of the left index finger* under the *right collarbone*, then the palm side of the *tip of the right index finger* under the *left collarbone*, followed by placing the palm side of the *tip of the right index finger* under the *right collarbone*.[12]

After the palm side of the index fingertip of each hand have stimulated

---

[10]Callahan refers to the TE-3 acupoint as the *gamut spot*.

[11]Callahan refers to the K-27 points as the cb or collarbone points.

[12]The order in which the K-27 points are treated does not appear to be important. The therapist may just as effectively conduct the procedure randomly.

each of the K-27 points, the same process is repeated with the *index finger knuckle* of each hand.

As discussed earlier, the palm side and back side of the hand have different electromagnetic polarities. Thus, the purpose of using both the index finger-tip and index finger knuckle of each hand is to stimulate the K-27 points in every possible combination of polarities, normalizing polarities front to back and left to right.

To summarize, the fingertip and knuckle of each hand are sequentially placed at each K-27 point while TE-3 is stimulated and the client proceeds through five breathing positions. The fingertip and knuckle positions are as follows:

1. left fingertip under left collarbone
2. left fingertip under right collarbone
3. right fingertip under left collarbone
4. right fingertip under right collarbone
5. left knuckle under left collarbone
6. left knuckle under right collarbone
7. right knuckle under left collarbone
8. right knuckle under right collarbone

Collarbone (K-27) Breathing Diagnosis and Treatment

In all, this procedure entails 40 separate treatments. That is, it involves eight K-27 stimulation positions *times* five breathing positions. While it is perhaps easy enough to do all of the treatments as outlined above, individual cases vary such that not all of the treatments are needed, and in some instances the necessary treatment phases appear to require more extensive stimulation than is achieved by simply tapping on TE-3 for five to seven times while holding a specific phase of breathing. Often more profound and enduring treatment effects are achieved by combining manual muscle testing diagnosis with these treatments.

As with the aforementioned treatments for neurologic disorganization, before conducting this protocol the results of manual muscle testing are found to be unpredictable and other signs of neurologic disorganization may be present. (It should be noted that often the neurologic disorganization is "hidden" and only becomes apparent during therapy localizing of specific phases of breathing combined with the various K-27 positions.)

The therapist begins by locating a strong indicator muscle. He/she tests the indicator muscle while the client *breathes normally* while touching the *left* K-27 point with the *right index finger*. If the indicator muscle remains strong, switching is not present at this location. If the indicator muscle weakens, either the therapist or client stimulates a TE-3 point (on the back of either hand between the little finger and ring finger) while the client continues to hold this position. The indicator muscle must test strong at this location before the examiner proceeds to evaluate other locations. In this way, the examiner and client move through the 40 combinations of breathing positions and stimulation points. It is not essential that they follow a particular order.

While there are other methods of diagnosing and correcting neurologic disorganization, I have described a fairly comprehensive list of accepted methods. Having a wide choice of ways to diagnose and treat this factor prepares the practitioner to assist clients thoroughly and consistently.

We now turn to another phenomenon which is related to polarity switching but requires more specificity and appears to be primarily and most fundamentally related to psychological factors: *psychological reversal*. Blocks arising from psychological reversal do not deter diagnoses, but they can prevent treatment itself from being effective.

Chapter 5

BLOCKS TO TREATMENT EFFECTIVENESS II: PSYCHOLOGICAL REVERSAL

The way out is through the door.
Why is it that no one will use this method?

— *Confucius*

PSYCHOLOGICAL REVERSAL, a term coined by Callahan (1981), refers to interference phenomena or psychological-bioenergy blocks, self-sabotaging states that occur when one's "motivation operates in a way that is directly opposed to the way it should work" (Callahan & Perry, 1991, p. 41). Psychological reversal has similarity to *Tibetan energy, figure "8" energy*, and *over-energy* (Rochlitz, 1995), as well as *reversal of the body morality* and the *umbilicus problem* as discussed by Diamond (1980a). These phenomena account for instances in which a person's consciously expressed desire is not met by his or her overt actions, indicating that the negative motivation resides at unconscious levels. The territory covered by these phenomena includes both pathologic as well as normal functioning. Thus, one can be psychologically reversed for being in an emotionally healthy relationship, for recovering from an alcohol or cocaine addiction, for being physically healthy, etc. It even applies to performance areas such as being able to excel at golf or tennis, assuming that the individual in question possesses sufficient athletic prowess to excel in the sport.

Diamond (personal communication, 1997), observing that unconscious motives can be at odds with one's expressed intentions, notes that the concept of reversal is really the essence of psychoanalytic thought. He also relates this phenomenon to the debates among students over the *Torah* and *Talmud*, reporting that when the debate appears to go incessantly in a circle, a student might exclaim, "Perhaps reversed!" Thereupon the debaters would go off in a more productive direction about the issue at hand. Concerning his version of reversal, Diamond writes:

> An even more serious situation is that which I call *reversal of the body morality* [emphasis added]. It is as if the indicators have been reversed, the red lights green and the green lights red. In this state a person will test that hate is good, and love is bad. Rather than being directed towards the problem, energy is now actively directed away from it. Thus no healing can occur. (Diamond, 1988, pp. 15–16)

In a similar vein, Callahan describes psychological reversal as follows:

> At times we all become aware that we are behaving in a destructive and hurtful way toward people we love, and yet we seem helpless to stop behaving that way. It is almost as if our willpower is suspended and we seem unable to do anything about it. At such times we are what I call psychologically reversed.
>
> When you are psychologically reversed, your actions are contrary to what you say you want to do. You might say that you want to quit eating when you aren't hungry, and in your heart of hearts you really do want to quit overeating. But in reality you are continuing to overeat. You are sabotaging your own efforts, you feel helpless and you don't know why. (Callahan & Perry, 1991, pp. 40–41)

Callahan provided an example of reversal with a client whom he treated for weight reduction. In view of the fact that treatment was unsuccessful, he conducted the *straight arm test*, isolating the middle deltoid muscle of her shoulder. When he had the client picture herself at her desired weight or announce her desire to be thin, a weak muscle response was obtained. By contrast, a strong muscle response was evidenced when she stated that she did not want to lose weight or pictured herself heavier and stated that she wanted to gain even more weight (Callahan & Perry, 1991).

How should we interpret this and similar findings? Some might conclude that clients who demonstrate such results *do not really want* to achieve their stated goal. At times this may be correct, although it would seem that the lack of resolve, or resolve in the opposite direction, exists at unconscious rather than conscious levels. This interpretation is consistent with psychoanalytic findings, including parapraxes such as slips of the tongue, as well as a whole range of psychodynamic phenomena. "What the client says is so, is not."

It may also be suggested that the prospect of achieving a desired goal or the fear of not being able to achieve it produces significant stress that works against the client's being able to achieve the desired outcome, this stress also being reflected in the weak muscle response. The lower level of stress associated with the thought of not achieving the desired goal produces quite the opposite effect in the tested muscle and so does not impair its performance. Other interpretations are feasible.

There is an obvious incongruity when a person is reversed. The individual is blocked from fulfilling his or her consciously expressed goal, in whatever context the reversal operates. Moreover, psychotherapeutic results cannot be achieved when the client is reversed. This situation is not invariably equivalent to *secondary gains* in the traditional sense of the term, that is, the client being disinclined to improve due to his or her conscious or unconscious perception of benefiting from the "undesirable" state of affairs and being disadvantaged by "improvement."

Psychological reversal entails a level of self-rejection; yet, Callahan has not defined psychological reversal in psychodynamic or cognitive terms. His position is essentially that the electrical or electromagnetic poles within meridians are actually reversed, and this is what prevents the person from fulfilling his or her expressed intentions. In his view it is this reversal of polarity, the electromagnetic substrate, that accounts for the self-sabotaging behaviors.

Another possible explanation is that reversal is a manifestation of the misinterpretation of sensory data.

> One possible mechanism underlying the phenomenon appears to operate at the perceptual level whereby sensory data are misinterpreted, yielding an opposite or incongruent affect or emotion to that normally experienced. Thus that which is negative for one feels positive when experienced in a state of psychological reversal, and is therefore engaged in despite one's conscious, cognitive understanding of its detrimental effects. (Gallo, 1998, p. 104)

Clearly, psychological reversal can be a manifestation of various interacting causes. While bioenergy invariably comes into play when one is psychologically reversed, the reversed polarity can be the result of severe psychological stress, structural misalignment, exogenous toxins such as allergens, various types of electropollution (Becker, 1990), nutritional deficits, conscious ambivalence, and even degrees of unconscious psychodynamics. Sometimes there can be conscious or relatively unconscious secondary gains or other perceptions that trigger the electromagnetic polarity reversal, which in turn serves to block the actualization of the consciously expressed goal. In such instances the polarity reversal would be relatively secondary. Other times the energy reversal may be the more fundamental cause. In other words, sometimes it's the chicken and sometimes it's the egg. In either case the energy system is acted upon either by some level of thought perception, which in turn feeds back on itself, or by exogenous or endogenous factors, which in turn affect one's thought perception and everything else.

DIAGNOSING AND CORRECTING REVERSAL

The remainder of this chapter covers the identification, diagnosis, and corrections for several types of reversal, including *specific* or *context reversal, massive* or *global reversal, recurrent reversal, mini* or *intervening reversal, deep level reversal, criteria-related reversal,* and *criteria-related global reversal.*

Context Reversal Diagnosis[1]

There are various types of psychological reversal. The most basic or commonly occurring type may be referred to as *specific* or *context reversal,* such as when a person is blocked from getting over a phobia, depression, etc. This type of reversal is observed when the specific problem does not respond to the treatment efforts. The diagnostic method involves testing the indicator muscle after having the client say, "I want to get over this *problem.*" Or, the statement can be more precisely stated: "I want to get over my *fear of crowds*" or "I want to be able to understand and effectively apply the information contained in this book." If a context reversal exists, the indicator muscle will test weak in response to any of these test statements. If a context reversal is not operating, the indicator muscle will test strong. The therapist can also

---

[1]Callahan has referred to this type of reversal as psychological reversal and specific psychological reversal. In deference to Callahan I refer to this phenomenon as context reversal, since it seems to be more precisely descriptive.

test the indicator muscle for an opposite statement, such as, "I want to continue to have this problem" or, "I want to keep this problem" or, more precisely, "I want to continue to have this *fear of crowds*" or, "I do not want to understand and effectively apply the information contained in this book." In these instances the presence of a context reversal will be signaled by the indicator muscle testing strong, and ruled out if the indicator muscle tests weak.

It is important to emphasize that if a client tests as having a context reversal, this does not mean that the client does not want to get over the problem. It simply means that the client has a context reversal that is blocking its resolution. In rare instances it may be necessary to assure the client in this regard, since it can be rather demoralizing and counterproductive, to say the least, for a client to come to the conclusion that he or she really does not want to get over the specific problem for which he or she is seeking treatment. Also, some clients tend to feel quite embarrassed, mistakenly believing that the therapist perceives them as not being truly committed to treatment. In the majority of cases, clients do not experience a problem with this or other test statements covered in this chapter, and the therapist's nonchalance is explanation enough. However, it is important that the therapist-examiner be prepared for instances when such reactions do occur.

Context Reversal Correction

There are various methods for correcting context reversal — or any other reversal for that matter. Substance approaches involve nutritional support with *Brain RNA Plus* (brain ribonucleic acid with choline and inositol) (Diamond, 1980b), *Rescue Remedy*, a concoction of five of the Bach Flower Essences (Walther, 1988), and/or MinTran or MinBall (Durlacher, 1994). Because these remedies are reported to be helpful in highly recalcitrant cases of reversal, it is recommended that they be used on a regular basis for a period of time.

Along psychological lines, Callahan reports that he initially focused on assisting the client toward achieving self-acceptance by having the client state an affirmation such as, "I profoundly and deeply accept myself with all my problems and all my shortcomings" (Callahan, 1985, pp. 59–60). This would often correct the reversal long enough so that other treatments could be effective toward alleviating the psychological problem. This is similar to Diamond's claim that various meridian imbalances can be corrected by employing certain positive affirmations (Diamond, 1985). Callahan eventually found that the effects of the affirmation could be enhanced by concurrently addressing specific aspects of the bodily energy system, through the acupuncture meridians. He discovered that it was especially useful to have the client stimulate the *small intestine meridian*, by tapping on the little finger side of a hand at SI-1 or SI-3, while stating or thinking about the self-acceptance statement three times. More recently, he has dropped the use of affirmations, simply having the client physically stimulate an acupoint. In part this appears to be an attempt to divorce his approach to therapy from cognitive theories, since a positive affirmation treats at least partially by way of cognition.

Callahan later reported that having the client vigorously massage a tender intercostal *neurolymphatic reflex* on the left side of the chest while stating the affirmation worked well to correct psychological reversal, especially when reversal tends to be recurrent (Callahan & Perry, 1991).[2] He has hypothesized that the neurolymphatic reflex approach to treating reversal works by draining toxins from the lymphatic system, and that elevated levels of toxins are frequently associated with psychological reversal. He has also opined that this may account for the effectiveness of treating reversal by stimulating the small intestine meridian, noting that the small intestine is a principal organ of absorption.[3]

So how is context reversal corrected after it has been diagnosed? In most instances the correction can be achieved by having the client tap on the little finger side of either hand at SI-3 or vigorously massage the neurolymphatic reflex on the left side of the chest (possibly on the right side as well) while saying (several times) a relevant affirmation such as:

"I deeply and profoundly accept myself even though I have this *problem*."
"I accept myself even though I'm *fearful of crowds* [or another specified problem]."
"I accept myself even though I'm finding it difficult to understand and effectively apply the information contained in this book."

---

[2] The neurolymphatic reflexes are located throughout the body, but especially between the ribs (intercostal), in the pelvic region, and along the spine. The reflex employed by Callahan is located between the second and third ribs on the left side, several inches away from the sternum.

[3] It should be noted that although the small intestine and the small intestine meridian carry the same name, the anatomical organ as identified in Western medicine and the traditional Chinese medicine designation do not wholly coincide on this account.

Immediately after conducting the reversal correction procedure, the therapist should test for the context reversal once again, so that both the client and therapist can be assured that the reversal has in fact been corrected before proceeding with treatment.[4] If the correction has not occurred, the correction procedure should be repeated. If correction does not take hold after three attempts, another level of reversal should be explored (see below).

Massive Reversal

When reversal encompasses a variety of contexts, infecting many aspects of the person's life, it is called *massive reversal*. Many areas of the person's life are in shambles, as commonly seen in patients suffering from addictive or severe personality disorders.

There are a couple of diagnostic approaches for discerning massive reversal. One involves a comparison between having the client place the palm and then the back of a hand over his or her head while an indicator muscle is being tested. The muscle should test relatively stronger in response to the palm-over-head position. If the reverse is the case, this is an indication of massive reversal. This indicator should be followed by a verbal diagnostic test for massive reversal, which involves testing the indicator muscle after having the client say, "I want to be *happy (good, wonderful, etc.)*" or, "I want to have a *happy (good, wonderful, etc.) life*." If a massive reversal is operating, the indicator muscle will test weak to these statements. If there is no massive reversal, the indicator muscle will test strong. The therapist can also test the indicator muscle for an opposite statement, such as, "I want to be *miserable (unhappy)*" or, "I want to have a *miserable (unhappy, lousy) life*" or, "I do not want to be *happy*." In these instances the presence of a massive reversal will be signaled by the indicator muscle testing strong and ruled out by the indicator muscle testing weak.

Again, let me emphasize that the presence of a massive reversal should not be interpreted as meaning that the client really wants to have a miserable life. This is merely a test statement. Otherwise why would the client be seeking treatment? It is true that some people "enter" treatment with other motives consciously in mind, but massive reversal is really a different matter.

---

[4]Treatment in this regard refers to procedures directed at alleviating the individual's subjective experience of distress while attuning the particular problem that produces the negative affect. The most immediate indication of treatment effectiveness is a reduction or alleviation of the distress at the time that the treatment is provided, with the intended goal of ongoing improvement.

Massive Reversal Correction

The correction of massive reversal involves having the client massage the previously mentioned neurolymphatic reflex or stimulate SI-3 while saying several times some variation of the following: "I deeply and profoundly accept myself with all my problems and limitations." Immediately after providing the reversal correction procedure, the therapist should again test for the massive reversal, so that therapist and client can be assured that it has been corrected before proceeding with or resuming treatment. If the correction has not occurred, the procedure should be repeated. If correction does not take hold after three attempts, another level of massive reversal should be explored (see below). It should be noted that in cases of massive reversal prescribing repetition of the treatment on a regular basis between sessions if often beneficial. Some therapists, depending on their orientation, find it helpful concurrently to recommend or prescribe oral substances that reportedly support reversal corrections, such as the Bach *Rescue Remedy* or *Brain RNA Plus*, which includes choline.

Recurrent Reversal

The term *recurrent reversal* was coined by Callahan. One example of recurrent reversal is when a client is being treated for a particular problem, the intensity of the symptoms is decreasing, but at some point during treatment symptoms resurge in intensity. For example, if the subjective units of distress (SUD) originates at a 10, descends to a 5, and then spikes back up to an 8, this may be indicative of a recurrent reversal. While the resurgence can be due to other factors, such as another problem or engagement of another aspect of the same problem, the recurrence of reversal can be determined by once again running a reversal test. For example, "I want to get over this problem," or perhaps more precisely with regard to this example, "I want this problem to get lower than an 8."

It should be noted that when recurrent reversal frequently interrupts the treatment, this can result in both the client and therapist losing faith in the treatment. In such instances it is crucially important to help the client correctly understand this phenomenon. In other words, the client needs to understand that the treatment is working, even though the results are being reversed by other factors. These factors may include the client's being exceptionally stressed or angry at himself or herself, militant disbelief in the treatment, and energy toxins. Sometimes discussion about the treatment, along with procedures directed at the most prominent stresses, will be necessary to realize effective results. If a client is distracted by disbelief in the treatment, the therapist needs to step back and attend to pacing and rapport issues prior to resuming the procedure being employed to alleviate the psychological problem. Recurrent reversal may also account for an increase of symptoms after the treatment session is completed and the patient has returned to his or her everyday activities. This can be due to any number of factors, including energy toxins (see Chapter 12).

Recurrent Reversal Correction

Correcting for recurrent reversal proceeds along the same lines as context reversal. Have the client massage the neurolymphatic reflex or stimulate SI-3 while saying several times some variation of the following:

"I deeply and profoundly accept myself even though I have this *problem*."
"I accept myself even though I'm *fearful of crowds* [or other specified problem]."
"I deeply accept myself even thought this *problem* keeps coming back."

Immediately after the client completes the reversal correction procedure, the therapist should test for the context reversal again, so that both can be assured that it has been corrected before proceeding with or resuming treatment. If the correction has not occurred, the procedure should be repeated. If correction does not take hold after three attempts, another level of context reversal should be explored (see below).

Intervening Reversal[5]

Callahan describes a type of reversal that is evident when treatment progress is interrupted or stalled, which he refers to as *mini psychological reversal*. Here we offer the alternative descriptor of *intervening reversal*. In this situation, the SUD may be steadily decreasing with a specific treatment, but then the decrease comes to a halt. For example, the client may report a SUD of 10

---

[5]See *Energy Psychology: Explorations at the Interface of Energy, Cognition, Behavior, and Health* (Gallo, 1998) for more detailed discussion of this type of reversal.

that decreases to and remains at a 5 after a period of treatment, with additional treatment having no additional effect on the SUD. The diagnostic method involves testing the indicator muscle after having the client say, "I want to get *completely* over this *problem.*" Alternatively, the statement can be more precisely stated: "I want to get *completely* over my *fear of crowds*" or, "I want to be able to *completely* understand and effectively apply the information contained in this book." If an intervening reversal exists, the indicator muscle will test weak. If an intervening reversal is not present, the indicator muscle will test strong. The therapist can also test the indicator muscle for an opposite statement, such as, "I want to continue to have *some* of this problem" or, "I want to keep *some* of this problem" or, more precisely, "I want to continue to have *some* of this *fear of crowds*" or, "I do not want to be able to *completely* understand and effectively apply the information contained in this book." In these instances the presence of an intervening reversal will be signaled by the indicator muscle testing strong, and ruled out if the indicator muscle tests weak.

Not to belabor the obvious, the presence of an intervening reversal does not indicate that the client really wants to continue to have some of the specified problem. The statement is simply a test to uncover the presence of the intervening reversal prior to treating it.

Intervening Reversal Correction

The standard correction for intervening reversal also entails the combination of an affirmation with tapping or otherwise stimulating SI-3 or the neurolymphatic reflex points between the second and third ribs on the left side of the chest (and possibly right as well). The client is additionally directed to say or think several times one or a variation of one of the following:

"I deeply accept myself even though I *still* have *some* of this problem."
"I accept myself even though I have *some* of this problem."
"I accept myself even though I am *still fearful of crowds* [or other problem]."
"I accept myself even though I *still* have a problem *completely* understanding and effectively applying the information contained in this book."

Immediately after doing the reversal correction procedure and before resuming treatment, the therapist should again test for the intervening reversal. If the correction has not occurred, the procedure should be repeated. If correction does not take hold after three attempts, another level of intervening reversal could be involved (see below).

Deep Level Reversal

Another type of reversal uncovered by Callahan has been referred to as *deep level reversal*. He observed that while some patients did not show an obvious psychological reversal, treatment was nonetheless ineffective. Thus a reversal at a deeper level was suggested. As compared to testing the indicator muscle after having the client say, "I *want* to get over this problem," the test statement for deep level reversal is, "I *will* get over this problem." Alternatively, the statement can be more precise: "I *will* get over my *fear of crowds*" or, "I *will* be able to understand and effectively apply the information contained in this book." If a deep level reversal exists, the indicator muscle will test weak in response to any of these test statements. If a deep level reversal is not present, the indicator muscle will test strong. The therapist can also test the indicator muscle for an opposite statement, such as, "I *will* continue to have this problem" or, "I *will* continue to have this *fear of crowds*" or, "I *will not* be able to understand and effectively apply the information contained in this book." The presence of a deep level reversal will be signaled by the indicator muscle testing strong, and ruled out if the indicator muscle tests weak.

Intervening Deep Level Reversal

There can also be an *intervening* or *mini version* of deep level reversal, as there is with context reversal. The challenge statement to the indicator muscle is varied as follows: "I *will* get *completely* over this problem" or, "I *will* get *completely* over my fear of crowds." If an intervening deep level reversal exists, the indicator muscle will test weak in response to these test statements. If an intervening deep level reversal is not present, the indicator muscle will test strong. The therapist can also test the indicator muscle for an opposite statement, such as, "I *will* continue to have *some* of this problem" or, "I *will* continue to have *some* of this *fear of crowds*."

As with other types of reversal, the presence of a deep level reversal certainly and hopefully does not mean that the client will not be able to resolve the problem. Again, in rare instances the therapist may need to reassure the client of the purpose of the test statement.

Deep Level Reversal Correction

The correction for deep level reversal is similar to other corrections for reversal, combining stimulation of an acupoint along with an affirmation. The standard acupoint is on the *governing vessel* at GV-26, directly under the nose. Any variation of the following affirmations may be used:

"I deeply and profoundly accept myself even *if I never* get over this *problem.*"

"I accept myself even though I *will never* get over this problem."

"I accept myself even if I *never get over* my *fearful of crowds* [or other specified problem]."

With regard to correcting the mini or intervening version, variations of the following affirmations may apply:

"I deeply and profoundly accept myself even *if I never* get *completely* over this *problem.*"

"I accept myself even though I *will never* get *completely* over this problem."

"I accept myself even if I *never* get *completely over* my *fear of crowds* [or other specified problem]."

As always, immediately after providing the reversal correction procedure and before resuming treatment, the therapist should test for the deep level reversal. If the correction has not occurred, the procedure should be repeated. If correction does not take hold after three attempts, another level of reversal, perhaps a *criteria-related reversal*, could be involved.

Criteria-Related Reversal

Several years ago I was treating a client who was not responding positively to energy treatment. He was experiencing severe guilt due to a misdeed, even though he had turned his life around. Despite our attempts to correct for psychological reversals, the SUD level remained high and immovable. This aroused my curiosity, so I asked the client what he thought might be interfering with our success. "Maybe I don't think I deserve to get over this," he responded.

As a result of the client's report, it was possible to discern a different type of reversal, one that suggested the incorporation of a criterion in the reversal.

This appeared to be similar to deep level reversal in some respects, if we can take the test and treatment phrases for that level of reversal to tap into a criteria. At that time I directed the client to tap under his bottom lip on the *central vessel*[6] (CV-24) while saying aloud three times, "I deeply accept myself even though I *don't deserve* to get over this problem." After we resumed the specific treatments that had not worked to reduce guilt feelings prior to introducing the reversal treatment, the distress level immediately began to decrease.

At the time I referred to this as *shame level reversal*, since it seemed that the client's sense of shame was blocking the treatment efforts. The term has since been changed to *deservedness reversal* to more specifically reflect the criterion involved. Since that time a variety of other similar types of reversal have been identified, and attention to them has improved the success rate of therapy in my and other clinicians' experience. Durlacher (1994) has independently reported similar findings.

The interesting thing about these reversals is that they appear to be activated by or intertwined with criteria, and thus in general they are referred to as *criteria-related reversals*. For example, in addition to *deserving*, criteria such as *safety, possibility*, and *motivation* may be involved. The criteria can be applied to specific contexts or across several contexts. In the specific area, for example, a client may test that he or she will not get over a problem, does not deserve to get over it, or cannot get over it and be safe. These conscious or unconscious factors can interfere with therapeutic results.

I have found these reversal distinctions, sometimes expressed subtly, in a variety of situations. Often the client tests that he or she does in fact want to get over the problem but does not respond to the energy treatments. Many clients who test without a context reversal nevertheless test in the negative to the statement, "I *deserve* to get over this problem." In such instances they test in the affirmative to either "I *do not deserve* to get over this problem" or, "I *deserve* to continue to have this problem."

Other blocks occur with regard to *safety* for self or others (e.g., "It is *not safe* for me to get over this problem"), *impossibility* of getting over the problem (e.g., "It is *impossible* for me to get over this problem"), or lack of

---

[6]According to Diamond (1985), the *central vessel* is associated with the emotional state of shame. With this in mind I directed the client to tap at this point on that meridian in order to restore balance and thus alleviate the sense of shame. Eventually I came to diagnose the meridian point involved in the reversal.

motivation (e.g., "I won't do everything it takes to get over this problem").
There are more examples later in this chapter.

Criteria-Related Reversal Corrections

The standard corrections for *criteria-related reversals* entail the combination
of an affirmation reflective of the criterion and massaging the neurolymphatic
reflex point between the second and third ribs on the left side of the chest
or tapping or otherwise stimulating relevant acupoints. Among the viable
options are SI-3, on the little finger side of either hand; GV-26, under the
nose; the central vessel at CV-24, under the bottom lip; and the kidney
meridian at K-27, under the collarbone next to the sternum. While the
therapist can experiment with these points, it should be noted that any
of these acupoints or neurolymphatic reflexes can be therapy localized to
determine which is the most effective for correcting the reversal in question.
This is covered in greater detail below.[7]

While stimulating an effective acupoint or neurolymphatic reflex, the
client is directed to say or think a relevant affirmation. The most common
criteria-related reversals are covered below, with some observations about
their individual relevance and occurrences. It should be noted, however,
that such reversals are possible with respect to any psychological problem,
even though some may be more common in certain contexts. In addition,
it should be borne in mind that, while these reversals are discussed here in
terms of the patient's "experience" of safety, possibility, and the other criteria
in relation to the problem being treated, this "experience" does not necessarily operate at a conscious level.

DESERVEDNESS

This reversal is among the most commonly seen of the criteria-related reversals. Common sense dictates that if a person consciously or unconsciously
holds the position that he or she does not deserve to get over a problem,
attempts to alleviate the problem will be met with considerable interference.
This reversal is common among trauma survivors, patients with eating disorders, and those who have violated closely held personal values and morals.

---

[7]In most instances the neurolymphatic reflex on the left side of the chest or SI-3, on the little finger
side of either hand, will facilitate the correction.

Diagnostic statement: "I *deserve* to get over this problem" vs. "I *do not deserve* to get over this problem."   ·

Treatment statement: "I accept myself even if I *deserve* to have this problem."

Intervening diagnosis: "I *deserve* to be *completely* over this problem" vs. "I do not *deserve* to be *completely* over this problem."

Intervening treatment: "I accept myself even if I *deserve* to have *some* of this problem."

SAFETY

If a patient experiences the problem as affording some level of safety, it will not easily be resolved. This consideration does not necessarily apply to situations that are truly unsafe or dangerous. This reversal is common among patients with anxiety-related conditions and even patients suffering from chronic pain.

Diagnostic statement: "It is *safe* for me to be over this problem" vs. "It is *not safe* for me to be over this problem."

Treatment statement: "I accept myself even if it is *not safe* for me to be over this problem."

Intervening diagnosis: "It is *safe* for me to be *completely* over this problem" vs. "It is not *safe* for me to be *completely* over this problem."

Intervening treatment: "I accept myself even if it is *unsafe* for me to be *completely* over this problem."

SAFETY (OTHERS)

Sometimes the resistance to alleviating a problem is related to the unconscious perception that someone else will be harmed if the patient no longer has the problem. For example, a patient with erectile dysfunction may experience concern that if he gets over this problem he would stray in his fidelity, thus threatening his marriage and creating an unsafe situation for his wife. Of course, while energy treatments may alleviate the block, therapy may need to address the inclination to stray and other marital issues as well. Being willing to work on this concern may prove a major aspect of alleviating the reversal. Note that when using the diagnostic and treatment statements, the term *others* should be replaced with the name of a specific other if known.

Diagnostic statement:	"It is *safe* for *others* for me to be over this problem" vs. "It is not *safe* for *others* for me to be over this problem."
Treatment statement:	"I accept myself even if it is not safe for *others* for me to be over this problem."
Intervening diagnosis:	"It is safe for *others* for me to be *completely* over this problem" vs. "It is *not safe* for *others* for me to be *completely* over this problem."
Intervening treatment:	"I accept myself even if it is *unsafe* for *others* for me to be *completely* over this problem."

POSSIBILITY

Some patients experience deep doubt about their ability to resolve the presenting problem, for whatever reasons. While doubt by itself does not signal a reversal, if it is deep enough it will be consistent with reversal.

Diagnostic statement:	"It is *possible* for me to get over this problem" vs. "It is *impossible* for me to get over this problem."
Treatment statement:	"I accept myself even if it's *impossible* for me to get over this problem."
Intervening diagnosis:	"It's *possible* for me to get *completely* over this problem" vs. "It's *impossible* for me to get *completely* over this problem."
Intervening treatment:	"I accept myself even if it's *impossible* for me to get *completely* over this problem."

PERMISSION

In many instances this criterion operates in conjunction with another, such as *safety* or *deservedness*. It is as if the energy system is saying, "I won't *allow* myself to get over this problem because it isn't *safe* to get over it" or, "I won't *allow* myself to get over this problem because I don't *deserve* to get over it."

Diagnostic statement:	"I will *allow* myself to get over this problem" vs. "I will *not allow* myself to get over this problem."
Treatment statement:	"I accept myself even if I *won't allow* myself to get over this problem."
Intervening diagnosis:	"I will *allow* myself to get *completely* over this problem" vs. "I will not *allow* myself to get *completely* over this problem."

Intervening treatment: "I accept myself even if I *will not allow* myself to get *completely* over this problem."

MOTIVATION

Diagnostic statement: "I will do *what's necessary* to get over this problem" vs. "I will not do *what's necessary* to get over this problem."

Treatment statement: "I accept myself even if I *will not do what's necessary* to get over this problem."

Intervening diagnosis: "I will do what's *necessary* to get *completely* over this problem" vs. "I *will not do what's necessary* to get *completely* over this problem."

Intervening treatment: "I accept myself even if I *will not do what's necessary* to get *completely* over this problem."

BENEFIT

Diagnostic statement: "Getting over this problem will be *good for me*" vs. "Getting over this problem will *not be good for me.*"

Treatment statement: "I accept myself even if getting over this problem will *not be good for me.*"

Intervening diagnosis: "Getting *completely* over this problem will be *good for me*" vs. "Getting *completely* over this problem will not be *good for me.*"

Intervening treatment: "I accept myself even if *completely* getting over this problem will *not be good for me.*"

BENEFIT (OTHERS)

Diagnostic statement: "My getting over this problem will be *good for others* [specify]" vs. "Getting over this problem will not be *good for others* [specify]."

Treatment statement: "I accept myself even if my getting over this problem will *not be good for others* [specify]."

Intervening diagnosis: "My getting *completely* over this problem will be *good for others* [specify]" vs. "My getting *completely* over this problem will not be *good for others* [specify]."

Intervening treatment: "I accept myself even if my getting *completely* over this problem will *not be good for others* [specify]."

DEPRIVATION

Especially in the treatment of addictions, the issue of deprivation may serve to block progress. When this type of reversal is diagnosed, a discussion around this issue is apropos. In addition, the patient should be taught to treat himself or herself for this reversal when urges arise. At times this reversal correction will be needed before other treatments are employed to specifically address the urge and the addiction as a whole. However, it has frequently been observed that the urge decreases after the reversal is corrected. This is not unique to addictions but occurs with a number of problems, the common factor being a decrease in the SUD upon alleviation of the reversal.

Diagnostic statement: "I will be (feel) *deprived* if I get over this problem" vs. "I will not be (not feel) *deprived* if I get over this problem."

Treatment statement: "I deeply accept myself even if getting over this problem is (feels) *depriving* to me."

Intervening diagnosis: "I will be (feel) *deprived* if I get *completely* over this problem" vs. "I will not be (not feel) *deprived* if I get *completely* over this problem."

Intervening treatment: "I deeply accept myself even if I am (feel) *deprived* if I get completely over this problem."

IDENTITY

Some problems are so deeply ingrained that they become an integral aspect of the person's sense of self. Narrative therapists make a distinction between the person and the problem and then set out to exorcise the problem via externalization reframes and relabels through language patterns (Epston & White, 1992). To some extent this is what reversal corrections and other energy therapy procedures accomplish, although energetic interventions are included in addition to language patterns. While it may be difficult for the patient to affirm the following energetic treatment statements with conviction, when employed they have nonetheless been found to be effective.

Diagnostic statement: "I will lose my identity (or an essential aspect
                               of who I am) if I get over this problem" vs. "I
                               will not lose my identity (or an essential aspect
                               of who I am) if I get over this problem."
Treatment statement: "I accept myself even if I lose my identity (or
                               an essential aspect of who I am) getting over this
                               problem."
Intervening diagnosis: "I will lose my identity (or an essential aspect
                               of who I am) if I get *completely* over this prob-
                               lem" vs. "I will not lose my identity (or an essen-
                               tial aspect of who I am) if I get *completely* over
                               this problem."
Intervening treatment: "I accept myself even if I lose my identity (or
                               an essential aspect of who I am) if I get *completely*
                               over this problem."

Criteria-Related Massive Reversal

Another type of reversal that appears to be activated by or intertwined with
criteria is what I call *criteria-related massive reversal*. The standard type of
massive reversal occurs across contexts and is manually diagnosed with
statements such as, "I *want* to be happy." The distinction with criteria-related
massive reversals is that criteria such as *safety*, *possibility*, and *deserving*
operate within the reversal. For example, a client may test that he or she
will not have a happy life, does not *deserve* to have a happy life, or cannot
have a happy life and be *safe*. These conscious or unconscious factors can
interfere with therapeutic results.

I have found these distinctions in a variety of situations. One case that
comes to mind is of a man in his early twenties whose approach to life
suggested massive reversal. He was dependent on alcohol and cigarettes, his
relationships were poor, he could not maintain a job, he was living with his
parents, and he was in a major depression. Convinced that he was massively
reversed, I tested him with the standard statement, "I want to have a happy
life." He tested strong. He tested weak to the statements, "I want to have a
miserable life" and "I do not want to be happy." I then checked an indicator
muscle response to the following statements: "I will have a happy life" and
"I deserve to have a happy life." Both of these statements resulted in a weak
indicator muscle response, while a strong muscle response was found to the
opposing statements of "I will not have a happy life" and "I don't deserve

to have a happy life." Correcting for these criteria-related massive reversals resulted in highly positive changes in this patient's life. Within days of the initial corrections he secured a job and started the process of recovering from alcohol dependence. Ongoing use of the corrections within the context of psychotherapy resulted in further improvements. I realize that this is merely an anecdotal report and that there were many factors involved in this patient's improvement; however, positive results did not begin to occur until after these corrections were made.

FINDING THE REVERSAL

Some examiners have found it useful to screen for reversals by challenging to a statement such as, "There is a reversal (or another reversal or other reversals) blocking the resolution of this problem." In this case it is wise to educate the client about the nature of reversals. A statement such as this should suffice: "Sometimes there is a block to the effectiveness of treatment. Basically it is something that gets in the way of the treatment working, and it is different from the problem itself. This is called a reversal. There appear to be various kinds of reversals related to issues like safety, deserving, etc. Often the presence of a reversal can be determined by simply having you say that there is a reversal and then letting me test your arm (or other indicator muscle)."[8]

DIAGNOSING THE CORRECTION SPOT

While in most instances reversal can be energetically addressed by stimulating SI-3 on the little finger side of either hand or vigorously massaging the neurolymphatic reflex point between the second and third ribs on the left side of the chest (and possibly the right side as well), for greater precision these and other treatment points can be diagnosed via manual muscle testing. This procedure involves simply testing the indicator muscle after the patient makes the positive statement (e.g., "I want to get over this problem," "I

---

[8]Some examiners believe that informing the client about psychological reversal is unnecessary. They contend that since the therapist knows what reversal is about, the therapist's contact with the client makes that information available to the client's energy system, neurology, unconscious, etc. An even more transpersonal approach might assume that knowledge about psychological reversal is contained within the collective unconscious and therefore accessible to the client and diagnosable through manual muscle testing.

deserve to get over this problem," etc.) while therapy localizing a treatment point. The treatment point that produces a strong indicator muscle is the treatment point of choice. Sometimes it is necessary for the therapist to touch the treatment point itself if its location is such that the patient cannot easily therapy localize it. In order of frequency, the common psychological reversal correction points are the following:

1. *small intestine-3* on the little finger side of either hand
2. *neurolymphatic reflex point* between the second and third ribs on the left side of the chest (and possibly the right side as well)
3. *governing vessel-26* directly under the nose
4. *central vessel-24* directly under the bottom lip
5. *kidney meridian-27* in an indentation directly under the clavicle next to the sternum
6. *triple energizer-3* between and above the little finger and ring finger knuckles on the back of either hand

UNIVERSAL REVERSAL CORRECTION

Some therapists have experimented with all-inclusive treatments for psychological reversal. They hypothesize that specification is not essential, that all reversals can be subsumed under one *universal reversal correction* or even possibly a *permanent universal reversal correction*. For example, possibly all reversals can be treated with statements such as the following:

"I deeply accept myself even if I continue to have this problem for whatever reasons for the rest of my life."
"I deeply accept myself even if this problem keeps coming back for whatever reasons for the rest of my life."
"I deeply accept myself now and each and every time in the future that this problem might be inclined to resurface for whatever reasons."
"I deeply accept myself regardless of any underlying issues that may block my resolution of this problem now or at any time in the future."

Nims (1998) has developed an interesting permanent universal reversal correction. His method begins by testing for psychological reversal about whether the client's subconscious mind is willing to use his comprehensive treatment algorithm. He first demonstrates his algorithm to the client and then muscle tests the client on the statement, "I can use this simple procedure to eliminate any problem that I ever choose to treat." He reports that about 50% of people muscle test negatively to this statement. The reversed client is then directed to gently rub the K-27 acupoints (i.e., under the collarbones) while saying three times, "I accept myself even though I have this problem."

After this temporary correction of the reversal, he then uses his single comprehensive algorithm to treat this reversal. He directs the following instruction to the client's subconscious mind and muscle tests afterward to determine if the subconscious mind has accepted the instruction: "Now, I am saying this to your conscious mind and to your subconscious mind. Whenever you are treating any problem, you are not only eliminating the emotional roots and the deepest cause (belief system) for that specific problem; you are also eliminating anything that would make you keep the problem, ever take it back, ever permit or passively allow it to come back, or ever be receptive to its coming back, in any way, shape or form."[9]

Nims reports that after he has treated reversal in this fashion, he never needs to treat it again. This is the only psychological reversal that he ever directly addresses in his treatments. He reports that he has never encountered an instance when a client's subconscious mind did not categorically accept this instruction. After this permanent universal reversal correction, Nims treats what others refer to as psychological reversals with the same single algorithm he uses for every other problem. He considers psychological reversals to be no different from any other problem requiring treatment.

In addition to the various ways of conceptualizing, diagnosing, and treating psychological reversal and neurologic disorganization, there are a number of ancillary procedures that are integrated with energetic treatments. These are covered in the following chapter.

---

[9]More information on Larry Nims's psychotherapeutic approach, *Be Set Free Fast*, can be obtained by contacting him at 1400 East Chapman Avenue, Orange, CA 92866, (714) 771-1866, (714) 633-5722, or e-mail at nimsl@primenet.com.

Chapter 6

BASIC AND
ANCILLARY PROCEDURES

There seems to be a kind of order in the universe, in the movement
of the stars and the turning of the earth and the changing
of the seasons, and even in the cycle of human life.

— *Katherine Anne Porter*

THIS CHAPTER FOCUSES on some distinctions among three energy treatment
approaches: *behavioral kinesiology* (Diamond, 1978, 1979, 1980a, 1980b,
1985), *thought field therapy* (Callahan, 1985; Callahan & Callahan, 1996),
and the methodology presented in this text, *energy diagnostic and treatment
methods* or *EDxTM* (Gallo, 1997b). It also covers the methodology and
rationale of procedures, such as the *nine gamut treatments, brain balancing
procedure, cross-crawl exercises*, rapid stress reduction techniques, including
the *floor-to-ceiling eye roll* and the *elaborated eye roll*, and *resonance locking*.

BEHAVIORAL KINESIOLOGY

While there are several meridian-based diagnostic approaches, behavioral
kinesiology, as developed by John Diamond (1978, 1979, 1980a, 1980b,
1985), was possibly the first to specifically utilize alarm points to investigate
the acupuncture meridians as they interface with emotional issues. This
method involves determining which meridian or meridians account for the
emotional disturbance and then providing relevant treatments, including
discussion related to the associated issues/emotions, affirmations, redecision,
etc. (see Gallo, 1998, for detailed coverage of this topic).

Diamond's approach entails conducting the *straight arm test*, which isolates the middle deltoid muscle, while the client therapy localizes various alarm or test points. Initially the muscle is tested *in the clear* in order to calibrate the muscle response. Assuming that the indicator muscle is relatively firm, the examiner proceeds with a series of therapy localization tests.

Initially the client or examiner therapy localizes the *thymus test point* at the upper sternum. If the indicator muscle remains locked in place, it is concluded that the thymus gland, the primary regulator of the acupuncture meridian system (according to Diamond), is strong, and thus at that point in time the client's energy system is balanced. If, on the other hand, testing the thymus results in a weakening of the indicator muscle, it is concluded that the energy system is compromised.

The examiner then determines which cerebral hemisphere is involved in the energy imbalance. To determine this, a test of *hemisphere dominance* is conducted by again challenging the middle deltoid muscle of the client's left arm, while the client positions the palm of his/her right hand in the vicinity of the right ear adjacent to the right hemisphere, followed by positioning the palm of the right hand in the vicinity of the left ear adjacent to the left hemisphere (see Figure 6.1). Whichever side tests weaker, as judged by a weakening of the indicator muscle, is the involved side. If the muscle weakens while the client positions the palm of the right hand off the left hemisphere, there is left hemisphere involvement, and the imbalance lies in one of the following *midline meridians: pericardium (PC),*[1] *heart (HT), stomach (ST), triple energizer (TE),*[2] *small intestine (SI),* or *bladder (BL).*

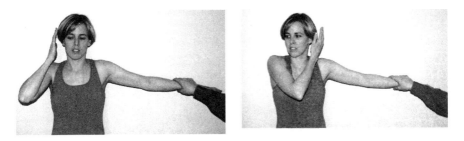

Figure 6.1 Test of hemisphere dominance

---

[1] In Diamond's system, the pericardium meridian is referred to as the circulation-sex meridian.
[2] In Diamond's system, the triple energizer meridian is referred to as the thyroid meridian.

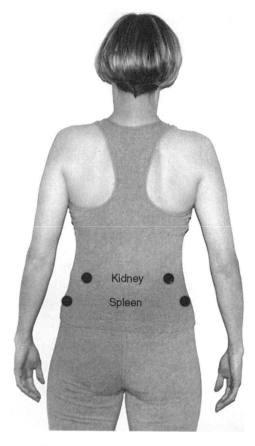

Figure 6.2a Alarm or test points

Alternatively, if the muscle weakens while the client positions the palm of the right hand off the right hemisphere, there is right hemisphere involvement, and the imbalance lies in one of the *bilateral meridians: lung (LU), liver (LR), gall bladder (GB), large intestine (LI), spleen (SP),* and *kidney (K).* The client then touches each of the alarm points for each of the meridians of the involved hemisphere while the therapist tests the indicator muscle. Whichever alarm point results in a weakening of the indicator muscle is the involved meridian (see Figures 6.2a and b for alarm points).

After the involved meridian is disclosed, the therapist might question the client about possible associated emotions. For example, if the lung meridian shows up, the therapist might question the client about possible chronic feelings of *intolerance* or *disdain,* emotional issues that Diamond believes

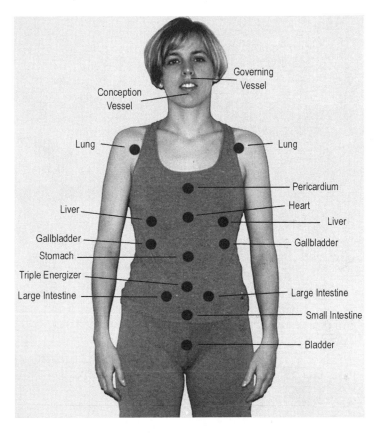

Figure 6.2b Alarm or test points

to be involved with lung meridian imbalance. After the client has identified issues, the therapist might have the client congruently pronounce an affirmation, such as, "I am humble, tolerant and modest." If this alleviates the lung meridian energy imbalance, the therapist again has the client therapy localize the thymus gland. If the thymus now tests strong, it means that the acupuncture energy meridians are now restored to balance. The client is advised to repeat the affirmation regularly to maintain balance. In time there should be a tendency for the balance to be sustained.

Alternatively, if the thymus tests weak after the lung meridian balance has been restored, the hemisphere dominance and alarm point tests are repeated in order to locate the next most relevant energy meridian imbalance. Perhaps next the large intestine meridian is revealed. This time the therapist might question the client about issues/feelings typical of the large intestine meridian: *guilt* and *low self-worth*. After the client has identified specific issues, the therapist might have the client congruently say an affirmation, such as, "I am essentially clean and good. I am worthy."

Possibly the next meridian to show up is the heart meridian, which may relate to issues such as *anger*. This imbalance might be treated with the affirmation, "There is love and forgiveness in my heart." This process is continued until the thymus tests strong, indicating that the energy system as a whole has been restored to balance. At this point the client would be advised to use the affirmations regularly. In time it is likely that balance will become the rule. Diamond also prescribes other therapeutic procedures, such as listening to or playing certain kinds of music, reading poetry, viewing specific works of art, etc.

At least in his early work, Diamond maintained that there was an order in which the meridian imbalances or layers emerged. In the above example, initially a lung meridian imbalance is revealed, followed by a large intestine meridian imbalance, and finally by a heart meridian imbalance. The order is lung → large intestine → heart. Emotionally the order is intolerance/disdain → guilt/low self-worth → anger.

Diamond points out that if the client is highly stressed at the time of testing, instead of a strong indicator muscle weakening when the alarm point is challenged, the indicator muscle will test weak from the start. In this case the therapist searches for the alarm points that strengthen the indicator muscle. This is referred to as *double negative testing*.

THOUGHT FIELD THERAPY (TFT)

Building on Diamond's acupuncture meridian testing procedures, Roger Callahan (Callahan, 1985; Callahan & Callahan, 1996) has specialized in double negative testing with alarm points being challenged while the client specifically attunes a psychological problem such as a phobia, trauma, addictive urge, depression, etc. He also maintains the idea of an order in which the meridians are diagnosed and treated, although his method involves having the client percuss or tap on specifically predetermined acupoints in the order, or more specifically *sequence*, in which they are diagnosed. Thus, if the sequence of meridians is lung → large intestine → heart, the client is directed to tap the following acupoints in the prescribed order: LU-11 → LI-1 → HT-9. Callahan refers to these acupuncture treatment points respectively as thumb → index finger → little finger, abbreviated as Th → If → Lf. (See Chapter 8 for locations of these and other treatment points.)

Callahan (1981) has also recognized the phenomenon of psychological reversal, advancing Diamond's notions of reversal of the body morality and the umbilicus problem. He has elaborated several types of psychological reversal (i.e., specific, mini, massive, and deep level) and delineated specific diagnostic tests and corrections for each. In addition, he highlighted the deleterious effects of neurologic disorganization and substance sensitivities, also referred to as energy toxins, with regard to treating psychological problems, and developed diagnostic tests and treatment approaches for these phenomena. (See Gallo, 1998, for detailed coverage of these topics.)

ENERGY DIAGNOSTIC AND TREATMENT METHODS (EDxTM)

Although the method elaborated in this text and elsewhere (Gallo, 1997b) is similar to those developed by Diamond and Callahan, it is different in many important respects. While all three methods involve the use of manual muscle testing to challenge meridian alarm points, and while an overarching order is evident, here it is not assumed or maintained that sequence of meridian points is relevant. Moreover, when several treatment points are needed in order to restore energy balance, the treatment points are diagnosed in a sequential order, but it is not assumed that they need to be treated in that order. While the cluster of acupoints may be important is such instances, it has been found that varying the order is of little or no consequence in terms of treatment effectiveness. It is likely that the treatment point order is an illusion created by the linear process by which manual muscle testing diagnosis is conducted. That is, since the examiner is able to physically diagnose only one point at a time, the process *appears* to be unraveling a precisely defined sequence. Actually, the energy disruptions in different aspects of the field are occurring simultaneously and the sequence is merely an artifact of signal strength.[3]

Another distinguishing feature of the method offered here is that many treatment points have been delineated for each of the meridians. Thus, while TFT, true to the methodology of therapy localization, invariably involves treatment of the stomach meridian at ST-1 or under the eye (e or ue) when

---

[3]This would be the case even if we were to have an electronic device that could diagnose the perturbations in a thought field. Assuming that such a device would reveal the perturbations, it might do so in a linear order, even though there is no true linear order fundamental to the thought field being diagnosed.

the stomach alarm point tests strong, EDxTM extends therapy localization and makes it more precise. The therapist-examiner has the client-subject therapy localize the treatment points themselves after the alarm point has revealed the involved meridian. Thus, an additional test is conducted in order to locate the most effective treatment point. In the case of the stomach meridian, this might be ST-1 (under eye or ue), ST-4 (corner of mouth or cm), ST-12 (supra-clavicular fossa or sc), or ST-45 (second toe or st). If none of these points tests strong, the examiner may explore other stomach meridian acupoints. This approach is consistent with ancient meridian therapies that recognize an array of acupoints, each with its own individual characteristics. Perhaps each point resonates a distinct frequency with its own unique characteristics in terms of emotional nuances, physiologic correlates, and such.

NINE GAMUT TREATMENTS

Partially based on findings by Goodheart regarding *eyes into distortion (EID)* (Walther, 1988), Callahan developed the *nine gamut treatments (9G)*. Goodheart observed variable muscle responses, depending upon the positions of the client's eyes. That is, a muscle might test strong while the eyes are directed straight ahead, but weak when the eyes are positioned lower left or lower right. Additional variations have been observed depending upon whether the client is humming a tune (nondominant hemisphere activity) or counting or multiplying (dominant hemisphere activation) or whether he/she is sitting, standing, or lying down, or engaging in different activities, such as walking, eating, etc. Consequently, Goodheart, after achieving therapeutic results, would increase the chances of their being maintained and extended by evaluating and treating the client in various EID and *body into distortion (BID)* postures. The six eye positions used by Goodheart are (1) eyes down right, (2) eyes down left, (3) eyes lateral left, (4) eyes lateral right, (5) eyes upper right, and (6) eyes upper right. These eye positions are consistent with those outlined in neuro-linguistic programming (Bandler & Grinder, 1975; Dilts, Grinder, Bandler, DeLozier, & Cameron-Bandler, 1979), each of which is assumed to access different brain functions and areas of the brain.[4]

---

[4]Mark Furman and I have explored these initial findings regarding eye accessing cues in greater depth by taking into account recent developments in neuroscience. See *The Neurophysics of Human Behavior: Explorations at the Interface of the Brain, Mind, Behavior, and Information* (Furman & Gallo, 2000).

Capitalizing on some of these findings, Callahan developed the 9G as a *fine-tuning* device that likely activates various areas of the brain so as to enhance the therapeutic results obtained by the *major treatments*, the TFT term for the various acupoints used to treat a particular problem. For example, after a trauma victim has been directed to tap the sequence of *majors* at the beginning of an eyebrow (eb), under an eye (ue), under an arm (ua), and under a collarbone (cb) the 9G is inserted, followed by repeating the majors (i.e., eb, ue, ua, cb). After tapping on the majors, the client's experience of distress associated with the issue being treated generally lowers. Frequently, after the 9G is completed, the level of distress lowers even further. However, since the 9G primarily serves to tune in other related aspects of the thought field for treatment, further lowering of distress may not be evident. Callahan states:

> The theory behind the gamut treatments is that we are balancing various functions of the brain with each treatment in regard to the particular problem we are treating. Each problem needs to be treated separately. It is as if the brain must be tuned to the right frequency for each problem for the treatment to work. (1990, p. 15)

When doing the 9G the client steadily taps between the little finger and ring finger knuckles on the back of either hand at TE-3 on the triple energizer meridian, referred to as the *gamut spot* in TFT (see Figure 6.3), while doing the following:

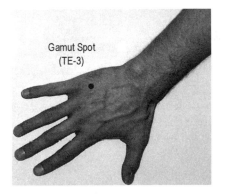

Figure 6.3 Gamut spot (TE-3) for nine gamut treatments

1. eyes closed
2. eyes open
3. eyes lower left
4. eyes lower right
5. rotate eyes clockwise 360°
6. rotate eyes counterclockwise 360°
7. hum a tune
8. count to five
9. hum again

Although some therapists prefer to simply take the client through the 9G after diagnosing the treatment points that collapse perturbations in the thought field, precision diagnosis and treatment call for specific attention to each of the 9G elements. That is, each of the nine treatments comprising the 9G can be individually diagnosed and treated accordingly. Some have concluded that the 9G is unnecessary, since immediate and sometimes resilient treatment effects are often evident after simply tapping a prescribed sequence of meridian points. However, if this conclusion is drawn in the absence of sound empirical testing, it is an uninformed conclusion that may lead to treatment failure, since thorough treatment may not be provided.

While the 9G can simply be inserted, as is done with TFT algorithms, one cannot be certain that the needed treatment effect has been delivered in this fashion. On the other hand, if each component is individually diagnosed and treated, and then diagnosed again to be certain that each component has been adequately treated, thorough treatment effects are ensured.

For example, after the treatments indicated through diagnosis have been provided, the therapist tests the indicator muscle while the client closes his or her eyes. The relevant thought field is still attuned (e.g., a phobia for dogs). If the muscle tests weak, the therapist or client taps on the gamut spot while the client continues to keep his/her *eyes closed*. After a few seconds of this treatment, the eyes closed position is tested again. If the indicator still tests weak, additional treatment is provided in that position. Once the eyes closed position tests strong, the client proceeds through each of the remaining 9G components until each tests strong. In this way a number of factors that can resurrect the problem have been addressed.

It should be noted that the three final treatments of the 9G are: *hum, count, hum*. Callahan contends that the order of these components is important. Sometimes diagnosis reveals that the client needs treatment in the second hum position, but not the first. There also seems to be a distinction between humming and then counting vs. counting and then humming. The essence of this distinction may be neurologically based, in that humming a tune is a more nondominant cerebral hemisphere activity and counting is a more dominant cerebral hemisphere activity. The directionality is also possibly relevant. That is, is there a difference in consciousness when the focus of activation is right hemisphere followed by left hemisphere as compared to left hemisphere followed by right hemisphere? Because of these and other implicit possibilities, each of these components should be diagnosed and treated separately.[5]

BRAIN BALANCING PROCEDURE[6]

After several years of using the 9G in treatment, I developed a distinct treatment which appears to achieve equivalent results. This treatment is referred to as the *brain balancing procedure (BBP)*. It is based on EID principles and other principles related to cerebral functioning as well. As with the 9G, it is best to diagnose the individual components before and after treatment to determine what is essential and if the treatment has produced adequate results. Also, this technique appears to tune in other aspects or holons of the thought field germane to the psychological condition. After diagnosing and treating the core meridian point(s) involved, the BBP is provided prior to further diagnosis. (See Chapters 9 and 10 for further details.)

The BBP proceeds as follows: While steadily tapping on the lateral edges of the eyebrows on the triple energizer meridian at the TE-23 points, the subject proceeds with the following treatments (see Figure 6.4):

1. Close eyes.
2. Open eyes.
3. Independently or assisted by following the therapist's fingers, move eyes

---

[5]The same effect is achieved if the order is varied to *count, hum, count*. With a client whose left hemisphere is dominant, *hum, count, hum* is equivalent to right → left → right, and *count, hum, count* is equivalent to left → right → left. Although there are some apparent differences, each combination contains the sequence of left → right and right → left.

[6]Developed by Fred P. Gallo. TE-23 can also be utilized instead of the gamut spot (TE-3) when doing the nine gamut treatments. Alternatively, the brain balancing procedure can be conducted by stimulating TE-3.

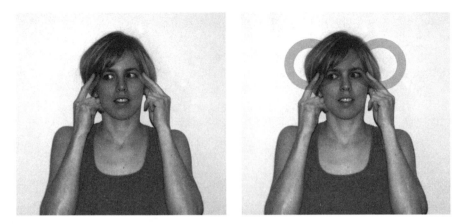

Figure 6.4 Brain balancing procedure

in a horizontal figure-eight (infinity sign). Continue the infinity sign tracking during the next three steps.

4. Count to or multiply by five.
5. Hum a few random notes or a tune for about five seconds.
6. Count to or multiply by five again.

CROSS-CRAWL EXERCISE

An offshoot of applied kinesiology and touch for health (TFH), *educational kinesiology (Edu-K)* (Dennison, 1981; Dennison & Dennison, 1987, 1989) entails the application of kinesiological findings to enhance learning and other areas of performance. This discipline includes a variety of *lateral repatterning* exercises, such as *homolateral crawl* and *cross-crawl*, designed to improve coordination of right and left hemisphere functions. While the procedures were originally derived from the work of Doman and Delacato (Delacato, 1966), Edu-K incorporates humming, counting, and specific eye movement patterns into the cross-crawl routines to enhance results in terms of improved attention and learning. Along with colleagues, I have also found this routine helpful for a number of children and adults with learning problems; it also adds dimensions that are not included in the 9G and BBP, specifically whole body movements, which are beneficial in some more difficult cases and especially delightful to apply in the treatment of children. The method can be used as a substitute for the 9G or BBP. Admittedly, it is rather difficult to directly diagnose the need for the individual components of the cross-crawl by muscle testing while the subject maneuvers the routine. However, after diagnosing the components of the BBP or 9G, the cross-crawl can be conducted, after which treatment effectiveness can be assessed again by diagnosing the components of the 9G or BBP. The cross-crawl exercises proceed as follows (see Figure 6.5):

1. Subject touches right hand to left knee after raising knee up from floor, drops hand and leg after touching, and then alternates hands and knees.
2. While continuing with this cross-crawl movement, subject regularly alternates counting to five and humming a tune for 10–20 seconds.
3. While still doing cross-crawl, subject visually rotates in a 360° circle clockwise and then counterclockwise, while continuing to alternate counting and humming for about 10–20 seconds.

STRESS REDUCTION PROCEDURES

The following procedures are often useful alone or in conjunction with other treatments. For instance, once a SUD level is significantly reduced with a single-point or multi-point protocol, one of the following stress reduction procedures may be employed to further reduce the SUD or to solidify results. It should be noted that these procedures can be used independently for stress reduction.

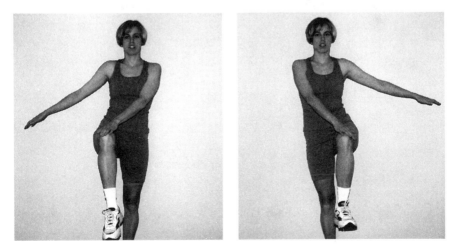

Figure 6.5 Cross-crawl exercises

Floor-To-Ceiling Eye Roll[7]

This procedure is conducted after the patient's SUD level is within the 0–2 range. The patient taps on triple energizer-3, located between and above the little finger and ring finger knuckles on the back of a hand (i.e., the gamut spot), while slowly and steadily rolling the eyes upward from floor to ceiling (see Figure 6.6). At this point the eyes are held at the raised position for a few seconds, and then the SUD level is reevaluated.

Elaborated Eye Roll

I and others have found that certain modifications of the basic eye roll serve to significantly enhance its effectiveness. This procedure, which is referred

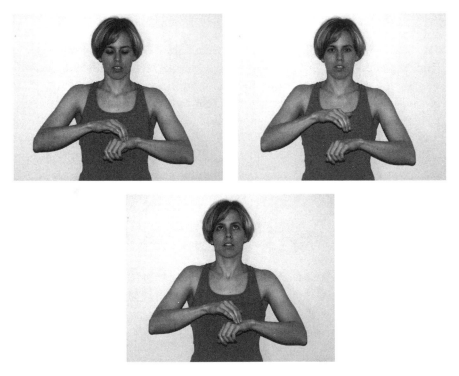

Figure 6.6   Floor-to-ceiling eye roll

[7]Developed by Roger J. Callahan (1990).

to as the *elaborated eye roll*,[8] is conducted after the patient's SUD level is within the 0–2 range, although it is also quite useful independently as a general stress reducer and as an adjunct for hypnotic induction. It proceeds as follows:

1. The patient taps on triple energizer-3 (G) or both triple energizer-23 points located on the lateral edge of the eyebrows (LEB) while slowly and steadily rolling the eyes upward from floor to ceiling.
2. While eyes remain at the raised position, the patient is directed to lower the eyelids and take a deep breath. Ideally, primarily the whites of the eyes show at this point in the procedure.
3. At this point the patient is asked to quit tapping and to exhale while lowering and resting his or her eyes in the closed position.
4. Generally a relaxing, floating sensation is experienced. The therapist may find it helpful to suggest that the patient "go with the flow."
5. Reevaluation usually reveals a significantly lowered SUD rating at this point.

RESONANCE LOCKING

Invariably treatment requires that the psychological problem be attuned during diagnosis and treatment. This can be accomplished in a number of ways. One approach simply involves having the client think about the problem and then assume that the energetic features will continue to resonate. In many instances this seems to hold true.

To ensure that the thought field remains engaged during diagnosis and treatment the therapist might intermittently remind the client to "think about it." In addition, *reminder phrases* can be employed during the treatment phase (Craig & Fowlie, 1995a, 1995b). For example, a client with a fear of flying can use phrases such as the following while tapping on relevant treatment points: *This fear of flying. Remaining fear of flying. Fear of crashing. Terrified of the take-off. Cramped up in the jet.*

Other ways to ensure resonance locking include the *leg lock* (also referred to as *pause lock*) and the *glabella tap*. These techniques appear to promote the locking in of "whole body information" without the client being required

---

[8]Thanks to Michael Galvin and Brian Grodner for alerting me to this highly effective variation of the basic floor-to-ceiling eye roll.

to consciously think about and experience distress about the issue being treated. This is of particular value when treating potentially highly distressing material, such as traumas, that tend to produce high levels of abreaction or even dissociative episodes.

The *leg lock* involves having the subject, while standing, turn his/her feet outward (e.g., Charlie Chaplin form) and abduct the legs, similar to what is done when assuming the second position in ballet. From a sitting position, the client can also effect the leg lock by sitting erect near the edge of the chair with legs and feet turned outward (see Figure 6.7). The leg lock is

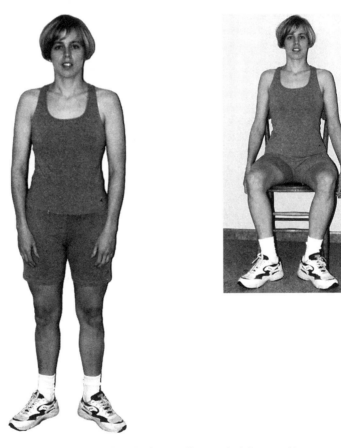

Figure 6.7 Leg lock standing and sitting positions

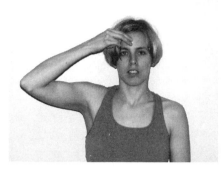

Figure 6.8 Glabella tap

introduced after the subject attunes the problem state, reports the SUD rating, and shows a weakening of the indicator muscle. At this point the weakening should remain as long as the leg lock position is maintained, even if the subject is not consciously thinking about or feeling anything about the psychological issue. The leg lock is maintained during the diagnostic phase as well as during the treatment phase.

Another way of sustaining a resonance lock is with the *glabella tap*. This procedure is introduced after the subject attunes the psychological issue, reports the SUD rating, and evidences a weakening of the indicator muscle. The client is directed to tap several times on the glabella, the smooth area between the eyebrows just above the nose (see Figure 6.8).[9] The thought field should remain attuned, even if the client is not specifically thinking about the issue at hand. This procedure does not require that the client assume any specific bodily position in order to maintain the resonance lock. It merely seems to extend the period of time that the resonance lock remains.

The procedures covered in this chapter are used in conjunction with other diagnostic and treatment methods presented in this book. They are

---

[9]This is also in the vicinity of the *third eye point*, which is located at *governing vessel 24.5*. This is also one of the four points used in the negative affect erasing method (NAEM), a method I have developed that is described in Chapter 7.

useful with regard to attunement, energy balancing, and stress reduction. Before delving into the specifics of precision diagnosis and treatment, we turn now to global treatments that have been found to be helpful for a wide range of problems. These procedures also serve as a useful introduction to the more precise diagnostic and treatment protocols that follow.

Chapter 7

GLOBAL THERAPEUTIC PROCEDURES (RECIPES FOR RAPID CHANGE)

> You were darkness once, but now you are light in the
> Lord. Live as children of light, for light produces
> every kind of goodness and right living and truth.
>
> —*Ephesians 5:8–9*

THIS CHAPTER INTRODUCES two global treatment algorithms that have been found to be highly effective for a wide range of problems, both clinical and otherwise: the *healing energy light process* and the *negative affect erasing method*. Using these therapeutic recipes can be a first step toward developing expertise with energy diagnostic and treatment methods at the more advanced and precision-focused levels. These procedures can not only be regularly incorporated into various phases of the overall treatment regimen, but also be utilized easily by clients themselves for self-treatment between sessions and for maintenance and treatment of problems that may arise after formal treatment has been completed.

THE HEALING ENERGY LIGHT PROCESS (HELP)

The initial and most simplistic algorithm is the *healing energy light process (HELP)*. It combines a number of treatment components in order to globally address the therapeutic issue or psychological problem. It combines some procedures from educational kinesiology/brain gym with the negative affect

119

erasing method (NAEM, described later in this chapter), diaphragmatic breathing, and an ancient yoga exercise of imaging healing light entering the body. At times acupressure holding is used instead of tapping on meridian and chakra points,[1] since touching is less likely than tapping to interrupt the meditative experience that is an integral aspect of HELP. In concert with this meditative feature, throughout the process it is recommended to the client that he/she not become attached to any intervening thoughts. Thoughts may come and go, but there is no need to become absorbed with any of them. This is a highly relaxing process that also generally corrects for switching/ neurologic disorganization and many levels of psychological reversal. The process is rather spiritually oriented as well, which appeals to some clients.

Aspects of HELP can be conducted with or without muscle testing diagnostics, if the clinician prefers. Although with experience the clinician and client may choose to streamline the process, in its more elaborate form HELP proceeds as follows:

1. Explanation

As with any therapeutic procedure, prior to taking the client through it, the therapist must explain the procedure and obtain permission to proceed. Assuming that the client is in agreement, HELP can be introduced with the following explanation or elements thereof:

I'd like you to imagine for a moment, if you will, that there exists a perpetual healing light. This light cannot be seen with our eyes, but it is the essence of all light. So anytime we see light in any form, we are witnessing this light too. And it is a healing light. It can heal anything as long as we open ourselves to its healing qualities, its healing powers. Now I'd like you to be willing to be open to such a possibility, even if you do not absolutely believe in the existence of the healing light. That is, if there were healing light as I describe it, would you be willing for its powers to assist in your healing? Would you also be willing for this light not only to heal you in the areas for which you are seeking assistance, but also to heal you in such a way that the problem will never come back in any way whatsoever?

---

[1]*Chakra* is Sanskrit for wheel. According to Brennan (1993), the chakras are in the shape of a funnel or vortex. Gerber provides the following: "An energy center in the body which is a step-down transformer for higher frequency subtle energies. The chakras process subtle energy and convert it into chemical, hormonal, and cellular changes in the body" (1988, p. 534). Both HELP and NAEM stimulate in the areas of the *brow* and *heart* chakras.

Each of the questions regarding willingness and intention can be subjected to manual muscle testing. If the client verbalizes "yes" and the muscle test is not consistent, further discussion and treatment for psychological reversal are advisable before proceeding.

2. Attunement

The client is directed to think about the problem for which he/she is seeking assistance. The person may do this in any way that works: visualization, self-talk, sensations, etc. However, it is neither necessary nor advisable for the client to access the issue to the extent that significant distress or abreaction occurs. It might be suggested to the client that he or she think about the problem only briefly so as to get a sense of how it feels. However, while many clients are able to observe a negative affect associated with the issue, not all are able to access much of a feeling. In these instances, perhaps the client has learned to repress the feeling aspects of the problem when it is not immediately present.

3. Scaling

If the client is able to observe a negative emotion associated with the problem, he or she is asked to rate the subjective units of distress (SUD) from 0 to 10. This may be further corroborated via manual muscle testing. For example, if the client reports a SUD of 8, the examiner would then have the client say, "It's an 8," after which an indicator muscle would be challenged. If the *muscular units of distress* (MUD) differs from the SUD, we tell the client that there is sometimes a difference between the emotional experience and the underlying energetic features of the emotion accessible via muscle testing. It should not be implied that the client was wrong in deriving a SUD, since this is certainly not the case. The person having the emotion is really the best authority about his or her own inner experience. Moreover, if the client were to feel demoralized to any extent for not being able to accurately estimate the "true level" of discomfort, this would introduce another negative emotion that would interfere with diagnosis and treatment. That is, another perturbed thought field would be intervening.

4. Imaginary Scaling

Rather than actually tuning into the distressing issue, the client can be asked to intuit what the SUD level would be if he or she were to attune it fully.

Generally the client has a pretty good sense of what the rating would be. This provides a baseline of sorts that can be compared with the client's more completely tuned in assessment of the issue after treatment has been provided. This approach appears to assist the client in accessing or attuning the perturbed thought field at a level sufficient for treatment, but lacking a signal strength high enough to produce a conscious experience of the negative affect. It might be argued that this procedure also adds a suggestive, positive expectation element to the treatment. This approach is recommended when the issue is highly emotionally charged, so that even the slightest period of attunement results in significant distress.[2]

5. Intention

Ask the client to hold in mind the purpose or intention for which HELP is being provided. For example, the process may be conducted to overcome a specific habit or addictive urge; to alleviate depression, anxiety, or physical pain; to resolve a trauma; or to enhance peak performance in a specific area. (The intention was initially addressed during the explanation phase and may, at that time, have been subjected to manual muscle testing.) Once the intention has been attuned, it is not necessary for the client to continue to think about it in a focused manner during the remaining steps.

6. Over-energy Correction

Next, the *over-energy correction* position is assumed as follows: The client crosses the left ankle over the right. Both hands are held out in front with arms extended and with palms facing. The hands are then turned over so that the thumbs are pointing down and the backs of the hands are touching. The right hand is then raised up and over the left hand, and the fingers are interlocked. The hands are then turned inward and up so that the interlocked fingers are resting on the upper chest, under the chin. The tip of the tongue is placed at the roof of the mouth behind the ridge at the center of the palate. Deep, slow diaphragmatic breaths are then taken in through the nose. It is helpful to close the eyes and center in on the slow, steady breathing. The client should imagine that the breath is coming in through the bottom of the feet all the way up through the body and then exiting through the bottom of the feet.

---

[2]This approach is similar to what Gary Craig, founder of emotional freedom techniques (EFT), has referred to as the *tearless trauma technique*.

7.   Healing Light

While continuing to breathe in this manner, the client envisions a perpetual healing light shining down from the heavens into the top of the head. This light should be a color that the individual associates with healing. One imagines that this light is traveling throughout the body, vibrating into every cell, every fiber of the body, from the top of the head all the way down the shoulders, down the back, into one's chest and stomach, into the legs and arms, into the feet and hands, into the fingers and toes. The light may also be seen as concentrating in the locus of the felt psychological distress or physical pain (e.g., head, chest, stomach, etc.). This phase of the process is continued for a few minutes to promote deep relaxation, even a fairly respectable hypnotic trance.

8.   Prayer Position

Next the fingers, arms, and legs are unlocked. The feet are set flat on the floor and the fingertips are positioned in a prayer-like position, the fingertips of the left hand touching the fingertips of the right hand. The palms do not touch. While holding this position, the client keeps the tip of the tongue at the roof of the mouth and continues to breathe slowly and steadily, inhaling and exhaling "through the bottom of the feet." He or she continues to envision the perpetual light glowing throughout the body. This position is maintained for perhaps a minute or two.

9.   Third Eye Point/Glabella, Under Nose, and Under Bottom Lip

Next, with light pressure, the index and middle fingers are placed at each of the following treatment points in turn, this position being held while a deep breath is taken in through the nose and then slowly exhaled: on the forehead between the eyebrows (i.e., the third eye point, also called the glabella), under the nose at governing vessel-26, and under the bottom lip at central vessel-24. If tension or discomfort is experienced, one imagines or thinks that the discomfort is dissipating. A statement such as the following can be made aloud or in thought at this and the following treatment points to embellish the effects:

"Any remaining discomfort is leaving my body, mind, and soul."
"Any remaining discomfort is leaving my whole being."
"I am eliminating any and all remaining discomfort attached to this problem."

10.   Thymus Gland/Central Vessel-20

Next all of the fingertips of either hand are placed at the upper section of
the chest on the sternum at central vessel-20 in the vicinity of the thymus
gland, and this position is also held with light pressure while a deep breath
is taken in through the nose and then slowly exhaled. Alternatively, the
client may lightly tap in this vicinity. Again, if tension or discomfort is
experienced, one imagines or thinks that the discomfort is dissipating and
this may be combined with one of the statements described above.

11.   Reorientation

Next the client's awareness is directed to the immediate surroundings and
he or she is given time to reorient comfortably. The presenting issue is
reconsidered. The client should be asked to focus on the issue fully and to
report a SUD rating, comparing this after-treatment measure with the pre-
treatment SUD rating or intuited SUD rating. This rating can also be
subjected to manual muscle testing for comparison. Most often the issue
has lost its negative impact.

   If the client does not experience a significant reduction in distress after
this process, we ask what he or she thinks might be accounting for this.
Listening to the client with an open mind can go a long way toward discovering why the process was ineffective. Perhaps the client was unable to focus
or thoroughly participate in the process because of some intervening issue.
Recognition and understanding of the issue should make a future attempt
with HELP more effective. Or, the therapist may learn that this approach
to treating the client's particular problem is entirely insufficient, and that a
more precision focused approach is needed. Several rounds of the NAEM
(see below) may alleviate the disturbance. More complex problems may
require the application of even more precisely directed protocols such as
the single point protocol, multi-point protocol (both described in Chapter
9), or core belief protocol (Chapter 10).

12.   Integrate with Discussion

If HELP proves effective and has been conducted as a part of a therapy
session, the therapist and client should now be able to discuss the psychological problem from a healthier and more relaxed perspective. Such a discussion can help to solidify the results realized from HELP. This phase often
yields meaningful insight, which is especially gratifying to clients who want

not only to alleviate their distress but also to reach a higher level of under-standing.

13. Repetition

The therapist and client may need to repeat HELP several times in order to realize substantial ongoing benefit. In addition, it can be prescribed as a homework assignment to be conducted on a regular, perhaps daily, basis. (See the end of this chapter for a client handout: *The Healing Energy Light Process: For Client Use.*) Usually this procedure is an aspect of or adjunct to a more comprehensive treatment approach. Often it is a useful means of initiating a therapeutic session prior to conducting precisely focused diagnosis and treatment. It can be helpful in closing down a session when the client has been experiencing considerable distress, since the HELP commonly alleviates stress profoundly.

NEGATIVE AFFECT ERASING METHOD (NAEM)

The *negative affect erasing method (NAEM)*, introduced elsewhere (Gallo, 1998), is a brief energy-based treatment that is clinically effective in treating a considerable range of psychological problems. It has been useful in the treatment of trauma/PTSD, specific and process phobias, various anxiety disorders, clinical depression, and a variety of affect-based conditions. Like HELP, this method can be conducted with or without manual muscle testing.

If the clinician prefers to provide NAEM without manual muscle testing, he or she can, after attending to preparatory issues such as rapport and explaining the method, skip to steps 11 through 18. However, if treatment progress is interrupted, this should alert the therapist to possible intervening blocks such as neurologic disorganization and psychological reversal. In such instances the therapist may attempt to intuit what is impeding progress or employ muscle testing to precisely diagnose the obstacles.

Below I present a comprehensive manual muscle testing algorithm. Prac-ticing diagnosis at this basic level is a useful introduction to diagnosis and an important step in the transition to the more advanced diagnostic and treatment protocols presented later.

1. Preparation

Prior to conducting NAEM, the therapist should address a number of prelimi-nary considerations, including establishing rapport, obtaining a thorough

history from the client, developing a comprehensive treatment plan, administering relevant questionnaires and psychometrics when needed, explaining
the purpose and method involved in energy diagnostics and treatment, and
securing permission to proceed in this manner.

While simply tapping on or alternatively stimulating relevant acupoints
is a useful technique toward resolving significant aspects of various psychological problems, in most instances it alone does not qualify as a sufficiently
comprehensive therapeutic approach. Also, approaching therapy in this manner might convey the mistaken notion to the client—not to mention the
therapist—that the *real cause* of the psychological problem is a disruption
in the body's energy system and that the client's only choice in the matter
is to stimulate acupoints in order to rebalance a bioenergy system that
somehow operates independently of or separately from the client. While we
maintain that there is a disruption in the energy system at such times, and
while it may prove highly efficient to treat the psychological problem by
directly addressing the energy system, it does not then follow that the energy
disruption is the real cause of the psychological problem. It only proves that
this is a highly efficient way to reduce, and in many instances eliminate,
distress, and it suggests that the energy system disruption is one of the
fundamental ongoing causes of the problem. To conclude otherwise is to
overlook the factors that sparked the energy disruption in the first place, as
well as the person's level of awareness, belief system, and choices that
maintain, albeit inadvertently, the energy disruption. One can also easily
argue that the client's level of consciousness and spiritual-moral development
are important factors in the genesis and maintenance of some types of
problems. In addition, we would be remiss if we were to overlook the
various systemic factors, such as relationships with significant others,
family, community, etc., and other environmental and various biological
factors.

Treatment must take into account all of these factors. Moreover, it is
generally important to inform clients about other important aspects of experience, such as the relevance of thought in the creation of experience and
how to achieve higher levels of thought awareness. Besides alleviating some
specific problems such as trauma and phobias, being freed of the negative
effects of certain thought fields creates space for a greater state of being and
development. Stimulating relevant acupoints to alleviate distress is akin to
giving the client the proverbial fish, as compared to teaching him or her
how to fish. While teaching the client when and where to tap is certainly
a move in the right direction, fostering higher levels of thought awareness

goes a step beyond, encouraging a philosophical shift that leads to a stable, healthy state of being.

2. Introductory Statement

Chapter 3 covers ways to introduce manual muscle testing. However, for the sake of convenience, here is an introductory statement for introducing NAEM:

There are many ideas about the causes of psychological and emotional problems. Some therapists and scientists say that stressful events in your life, negative thoughts, and even chemical imbalances contribute to these problems. Certainly this is all true, since all these things work together. Seldom is there only one cause for a problem. In fact, in addition to the others, it seems that there is an electrical part, a switch that turns on the emotional problem. So if there is an ongoing disturbing situation in your life or a terrible event or trauma that happened to you, you'll likely have certain thoughts or beliefs about it, and these thoughts will trigger electrical impulses in your brain and body that produce imbalances in your chemistry and upsetting emotions like anxiety, depression, anger, and so on. And this all feeds back into the whole system and keeps it going.

It seems that the electrical part of the problem can be diagnosed by using a simple muscle checking procedure. You see, the muscles and nerves work together, so when you have an upsetting emotion, it causes a change in your muscles, too. The muscles tend to become firmer with positive thoughts and emotions, and somewhat loose or weaker with negative thoughts and emotions. It isn't that the muscles are really weak at such times, just that the electricity moving through the nerves gets interrupted so that the muscle momentarily cannot operate at its best. The method involves checking the firmness in a shoulder muscle while you hold your arm out straight (or the muscles in your fingers as you make a circle with your index finger and thumb, etc.). I'll ask you to think about the problem that you want help with to see how this affects the muscle. I'll also have you touch certain places on your body that are like circuit breakers and test the muscle in response to certain statements. I may ask you to do some other things, like moving your eyes in different directions, humming, and counting. We really need to work together cooperatively in this if it's going to work. Would this all be okay with you?

3. Qualifying the Indicator Muscle

As discussed in Chapter 3, it is important to qualify the indicator muscle. Essentially, the therapist asks the client if it is all right to press on the arm while isolating a deltoid muscle in the shoulder (or apply pressure to whatever muscle is chosen). The purpose here is to screen for any contraindications to using that muscle, such as a physical problem. Obviously, it would be ill advised to conduct this procedure with a particular muscle if this could cause physical pain or possibly result in physical injury.

4. Preliminary Calibration Tests

Often it is useful to preface the diagnostic process by conducting a few preliminary tests or demonstrations of the muscle testing phenomena. For example, the examiner can simply ask the subject to "hold" and then press on the subject's extended arm.[3] Assuming that the subject is not attuning a distressing thought and is not touching anyplace on his or her body with the free hand, this phase is referred to as testing *in the clear.* This phase provides a baseline, a measure of the subject's ability to hold the muscle firm. After this phase, follow-up challenges can be compared to this baseline.

The subject can next be asked to state his/her name, prefaced by the statement, "My name is (*correct name*)." Again, testing the indicator muscle should result in a response similar to or firmer than the baseline. Afterwards the subject can be asked to state a false name, again prefaced by, "My name is (*wrong name*)." This time the indicator muscle response should be relatively weaker.

A number of other preliminary tests can be conducted with regard to what the subject ate at a specific meal, identifying the President of the United States, thinking about something pleasant as compared to something unpleasant, etc. Each time the subject's attention should be directed to observing and understanding the relevance of the muscle response.

5. Diagnosing and Correcting Neurologic Disorganization/Switching

If the preliminary tests are uncomplicated (i.e., a clear distinction between muscle responses is detectable), then the presence of neurologic disorganiza-

---

[3] For ease of discussion, from this point on the straight arm test (isolating the middle deltoid as the indicator muscle) will be used. It is recognized that this will not be the appropriate measure for some subjects.

tion is unlikely and the muscle response is adequate for making finer diagnostic determinations. On the other hand, if it is difficult or impossible to discern between weak and strong muscle responses, then this should be investigated further and corrected; otherwise, it will not be possible to accurately discern muscle response and diagnostic information will be obscured. (See Chapter 4 for further details.)

6. *Diagnosing and Correcting Massive Psychological Reversal*

After neurologic disorganization has been evaluated and, if present, adjusted, the examiner determines if a massive psychological reversal (MPR) is present. To review, MPR is a reversal across many contexts in the person's life, so that there is a tendency toward considerable self-sabotaging. This may or may not be relevant in the specific area for which the client is seeking therapy, although massively reversed clients can often benefit from more extensive treatment, even if they are presenting for only a delimited issue such as a specific phobia or addiction to chocolate.

The hand-over-head test also screens for MPR. If the client's indicator muscle tests strong when the palm is positioned over the head and weak when the back of the hand is positioned over the head, both neurologic disorganization and MPR can be ruled out in most instances. This test evidences few false negatives but more false positives; therefore, when the test suggests MPR, it should invariably be followed up with a more sensitive test. Specifically, the indicator muscle should be challenged while having the subject say, "I want to be happy" or "I want to have a happy life." If the indicator muscle tests "weak" in response to these statements, suggesting MPR, the muscle should again be challenged to the opposite statement, "I want to be unhappy (or miserable)" or "I want to have an unhappy (or miserable) life." In these instances, a "strong" muscle response is consistent with MPR.[4] If the client evidences MPR, that should be corrected following the procedure outlines in Chapter 5.

7. *Accessing the Problem State*

If the client is not neurologically disorganized, it is possible to detect when the problem is attuned. The examiner simply asks the subject to "think

---

[4]In addition to testing for and correcting MPR, the examiner may find it necessary to address criteria-related MPRs (see Chapter 5).

about" the problem. It is not absolutely necessary that the subject visualize the problem, although some may find this an effective way to attune at a high signal strength level. After the subject acknowledges that the problem is attuned, he/she is then asked to "hold," after which the indicator muscle is challenged. In a majority of cases the indicator muscle will not remain as firm as it was when tested in the clear, thus confirming that the problem thought field is attuned.

8.   Scaling

It is generally helpful to obtain a SUD rating, either before or after challenging the indicator muscle, while the perturbed thought field is attuned. The examiner might simply ask, "As you think about the problem (e.g., phobia, trauma, depression) at this very moment, on a scale of 0–10, with 10 being the highest level of discomfort and 0 being no discomfort at all, how much discomfort do you feel?" After the subject offers a number, the SUD can be further corroborated by challenging the indicator muscle. Although the indicator muscle will usually test "weak" (off) when the problem state is attuned, it will test "strong" (on) when the actual rating (0–10) is stated. In most cases the SUD and muscular ratings will be equivalent; however, when they do not coincide, the examiner and subject can determine the precise muscular rating via muscle testing. Specifically, the subject states various ratings and the examiner challenges the muscle each time. For example, the subject says, "It's a 5," after which the examiner challenges the indicator muscle. If the muscle remains firm, the rating is accepted as accurate; if the muscle becomes slack, the rating is rejected and another rating is tested. This procedure assists the client and examiner in obtaining an accurate baseline upon which to assess progress toward the goal of alleviating emotional distress. When there is a difference between the stated SUD and the rating obtained by muscle testing, the therapist might inform the client that, while there is a variation, the client is really the best authority on how he/she feels. It might also be pointed out that the distinction here is one between how the client feels (i.e., SUD rating) and the energetic structure underlying the problem (i.e., muscular response) for which treatment is desired.[5]

---

[5]The therapist should not induce any feelings of shame by incorrectly suggesting that the client is wrong in his/her SUD rating.

Some practitioners choose not to obtain a SUD rating; instead, they simply accept qualitative statements from the client. While this will not necessarily affect treatment effectiveness, a considerable amount of potentially useful information is lost. Precise estimates of treatment progress will be indiscernible. For example, a rating of 10 followed by a rating of 5 and then one of 2, is different from the "equivalent" ratings of: "It bothers me a lot . . . , It bothers me less . . . , It doesn't bother me now." The SUD rating assists the client and therapist in making fine distinctions.

It is also possible that application of a SUD-free approach on a regular basis will more frequently incur instances of what Callahan has referred to as the *apex problem* (Gallo, 1998). For instance, if the client provides a rating of 10 and then later reports a rating of 1, it is difficult to doubt that improvement has occurred; a qualitative rating, on the other hand, can be questioned and dismissed.

9. Resonance Locking

After the perturbed thought field has been attuned, in most instances it will continue to resonate for a period of time sufficient for the completion of the diagnostic and therapeutic procedures. This suggests a kind of *entrainment* or *resonance lock* that can be described in terms of a reverberating of the energetic aspects of the problem state or perhaps in terms of subconscious awareness. No doubt, a neurologic and chemical component is also involved in the experience. Regardless of how this is conceptualized, we know that when we think about something either positive or negative, the feelings or affects associated with the thought continue to linger for a period of time even after the thought has been consciously dismissed.

Even though this resonating effect is likely, in some instances we cannot be sure that there is signal strength sufficient for proper diagnosis of the energetic aspects of the problem. This may be a function of the degree to which the client is able to consciously access the thought field, or perhaps it speaks of his or her skill at repression. This problem can be overcome by employing a simple *resonance locking procedure*, such as the *leg lock* (also referred to as *pause lock*) or the *glabella tap* (see pp. 115–118). Both of these procedures appear to promote the locking in of "whole body information" without the client's being required to consciously think about and experience distress about the issue being treated. This is of particular value when treating potentially highly distressing material such as traumas, which tend to produce high levels of abreaction or even dissociative episodes.

10. Diagnosing and Correcting Specific Psychological Reversal

Now that the psychological issue is attuned and locked in, the examiner can test for and correct psychological reversals that could block the progress of treatment, as described in Chapter 5.

11. Diagnosing and Correcting Other Reversals

Next the therapist may wish to rule out alternative reversals, including deep level and criteria-related reversals. The same procedures and principles apply in these areas and are described in Chapter 5.

12. NAEM Treatment Points

There are four primary NAEM treatment points (see Figure 7.1). The same points are used to treat any and all psychological problems:

TE = third eye point, between the eyebrows. This is the GV-24.5 point on the governing vessel and it is also the section of the forehead called the glabella.

UN = under nose. This point is also on the governing vessel at GV-26. This point is used in applied kinesiology to treat neurologic disorganization.

UL = under bottom lip. This point is on the central vessel at CV-24. This point is also used in applied kinesiology to treat neurologic disorganization.

CH = chest. This point is also on the central vessel in the vicinity of CV-20, which is also over the thymus gland.

13. Stimulating Treatment Points

After the specific issue has been attuned, the client is directed to stimulate each of the treatment points for approximately five seconds. The usual order of stimulation is as follows: TE → UN → UL → CH. In the standard method the client taps on the treatment point with the tips of his/her fingers. Other means of stimulation include pressing or rubbing on each of the points for several seconds. Some clients prefer these alternative methods or experience physical pain at the treatment point location with tapping.

When clients do not respond adequately to the TE → UN → UL → CH order, varying the order of points has been found to be effective. The next

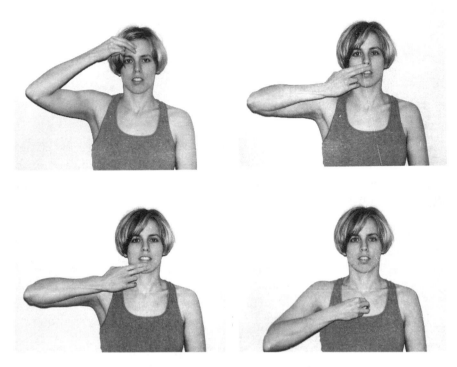

Figure 7.1 NAEM treatment points

most common order is UN → UL → TE → CH. When this works, it is likely that the client was in a state of neurologic disorganization, and stimulating the governing and central vessel points (i.e., UN and UL) alleviated the condition so that the specified purpose of the treatment could achieve results. It should be noted that repeating the TE → UN → UL → CH order several times will often produce results even without adjusting the stimulation sequence.

Another highly effective way of conducting this treatment is to ask the client to stimulate the TE point and report when he or she observes the SUD level beginning to descend. As soon as a decrease is acknowledged, the therapist intermittently requests SUD ratings while the client continues to stimulate the acupoint. Once there is a significant decrease in the SUD rating, the therapist directs the client to stimulate the other NAEM points.

When the results from stimulating the NAEM treatment points are insufficient, the effects may be enhanced by having the client place the palm of his or her free hand on the occipital region at the back of the head, in the vicinity of governing vessel-17, while placing the tongue against the palate approximately one inch behind the teeth. This position is held while the various NAEM treatment points are stimulated.

14.   Ongoing Evaluation

Intermittently the therapist may wish to take a SUD rating, sometimes corroborated by manual muscle testing.[6] If the SUD has decreased by at least two points with each evaluation, stimulation of the NAEM treatment points is resumed until the SUD reaches zero or stops decreasing.

If the SUD rating stops decreasing, the therapist should check for and correct any intervening reversal before continuing stimulation. Callahan (1985) calls these intervening reversals *mini reversals*. Possible reversals at this point include the intervening version of specific reversal (i.e., "I want to be *completely* over this problem") or any alternative criteria-related reversal (e.g., deserving, safety, possibility, motivation, deprivation).

If a specific intervening reversal is not revealed, the therapist may choose to check for the most common criteria that may block treatment progress, trust his/her intuition, or evaluate with a screening statement such as, "There is a reversal blocking the resolution of this problem." If testing this statement suggests than an intervening reversal is present, the therapist can explore various options. It is, of course, advisable that subjects have a basic understanding of what reversal entails. (See Chapter 5 for detailed coverage on reversals.)

15.   Balancing Procedures

When the SUD rating has reached zero, or has stopped decreasing without a reversal being involved, one of the balancing procedures can be introduced. These include the nine gamut treatments, brain balancing procedure, and cross-crawl exercises, as described in Chapter 6. While the therapist can

---

[6] For example, if a SUD of 5 is reported, the therapist can check further by challenging the indicator muscle after the client says, "I'm now at a 5." If the muscle tests strong, this further corroborates the rating. If the muscle does not hold firm, other ratings are tested. Ratings that do not coincide are seldom off by more than two points in either direction.

provide one of these procedures without bothering to diagnose its necessity, diagnosis both suggests which elements of the respective procedure are needed and verifies that the requirements of the individual elements have been fulfilled. Diagnosis may also inform the examiner that none of these procedures is necessary. It should be noted that conducting elements of these procedures (i.e., specific eye positions, humming, cross-crawl, etc.) is a way to assess and insure the thoroughness of the treatment effects up to this point. (See Chapter 6 for detailed coverage of *eyes into distortion (EID)* and related phenomena.) It should also be noted that the balancing procedures frequently tune in related energetic aspects of the thought field, making those aspects available for diagnosis and treatment.

16. Reevaluation and Further Treatment

After a balancing procedure has been provided, the therapist once again checks the SUD rating and sometimes corroborates it via muscle testing. If the SUD is not at 0, and a reversal is not present, stimulation of the NAEM treatment points is resumed.

17. Eye Roll Procedures

When the SUD is within the 1–2 range, the therapist may introduce either the floor-to-ceiling eye roll (ER) or the elaborated eye roll (EER) in order to reduce the stress level to 0. One of these procedures can be provided for "good measure" to insure that all traces of stress have been removed (see Chapter 6 for details).

18. Evidence of Bioenergy Balance

The indicator muscle generally weakens when a perturbed thought field is attuned. In most instances, after the psychological problem has been thoroughly treated, the client will observe a complete absence of distress when thinking about the issue (i.e., a SUD of 0), the indicator muscle will remain strong when attuning the thought field, and conducting the hemisphere dominance test will reveal a strong indicator muscle while evaluating either hemisphere (see Chapter 6).

As noted, in some instances the client does not experience any distress while initially attuning the problem, even though the indicator muscle generally weakens when the perturbed thought field is attuned. With thor-

ough treatment, the indicator muscle will remain strong while the client
again thinks about the issue. At this point it will also remain firm during
the hemisphere dominance test.

In some cases the client continues to report some level of discomfort,
even though both manual muscle testing and the hemisphere dominance
test indicate that the problem is resolved. Often there is a delayed experiential
effect and the subjective experience catches up to the energetic changes
within a few minutes. It may prove comforting to the client to be advised
of this effect.

19. Belief Instillation

After NAEM has alleviated the psychological problem, the client may spontaneously report a shift to a positive cognition or belief about the issue. This
makes sense, since negative beliefs appear to be affect-driven. Once the
negative affect is discharged, the negative belief often dissipates and is replaced by a positive cognition or appraisal of the situation. When such a
transformation does not spontaneously occur to the satisfaction of both
therapist and client, having the client rehearse an antithetical positive cognition while doing NAEM will help to solidify and enhance results.[7] For
example, a rape victim may have "decided" at the time of the trauma that
she was "powerless." After alleviating the trauma, one might ask her to hold
in mind a positive statement of her own choosing, such as "I'm strong and
I survived," while repeating the NAEM process. With a client who has been
treated for fear of flying, the combination of NAEM and a positive affirmation,
such as "I fly with comfort and enjoyment," might be used to instill the
associated belief. The degree to which the belief is incorporated by the client
can be gauged by using a 0–10 belief score, 0 representing a complete
absence of the desired belief and 10 representing the highest level attainable.
The goal is to elevate the belief score to the 8–10 range.

20. In Vivo NAEM

Between sessions clients can use NAEM in vivo. Many clients experience
this self-treatment to be quite empowering. The handout at the end of this

---

[7] Alternatively having the client tap on triple-energizer-3 between the third and fourth fingers on
the back of either hand (i.e., gamut spot), while rehearsing the positive belief will frequently achieve
similar results.

chapter is given to clients for between-session application and as a resource that can be used after therapy has ended.

Validation

The proof of this method takes place in everyday life. Even though it frequently results in a change within the desired context, only time will tell. Often, when the therapeutic results cannot be sustained, it is the result of other aspects of the problem that need to be addressed with this protocol. For example, agoraphobia is a complex anxiety disorder, with many aspects. If NAEM were to alleviate only a couple of these aspects, the problem would not be resolved; cure would involve neutralizing all of the anxieties and possibly even adding enjoyment in the previously anxiety-provoking contexts.

Now that globally oriented protocols have been covered, we turn to a compendium of the alarm (test) points and treatment points most frequently employed in energy diagnostic and treatment methods. These points are essential to the precision diagnostic and treatment protocols that follow.

The Healing Energy Light Process: For Client Use
© 1999 by Fred P. Gallo, Ph.D.

The *healing energy light process (HELP)* is a highly effective procedure that helps to eliminate negative emotional responses in a number of areas. It can be used to reduce anxiety, tension, anger, guilt and shame feelings, depression, fatigue, and physical pain, and to assist in the treatment of any other problems that you and your therapist have identified as appropriate for this method. You can use this process between sessions as directed by your therapist to assist in your overall treatment. Throughout the process you should not become attached to any intervening thoughts. Thoughts will come and go, but there is no need to become absorbed with any of them. HELP is usually quite relaxing.

1. Begin by having in mind the purpose for which you are receiving *HELP*. Hold your intention in mind. For example:

    My intention in doing this is to overcome depression.
    I am doing this to increase my confidence and comfort in social situations.
    I am doing this to eliminate panic attacks.
    I am doing this to eliminate this migraine.
    My intention in doing this is to improve my golf game.

2. Cross your left ankle over your right. Hold your hands out in front of you, arms extended, with palms facing. Turn your hands over so your thumbs point down and the back of the hands are touching. Raise your right hand up and over your left hand, and interlock the fingers. Turn your hands in and up so that your hands are resting on your chest under your chin.

3. Now place the tip of your tongue at the roof of your mouth behind that little ridge at the center of the palate. Take some slow, deep diaphragmatic breaths in through your nose. You might like to close your eyes and just center in on your steady, slow breathing. Also imagine that the breath is coming in through the bottom of your feet all the way up through your body. As you exhale, the breath is also exiting through the bottom of your feet. Comfortably hold in mind your intention while doing this.

4. While you continue to breathe in this manner, imagine that there is a perpetual healing light shining down from the heavens onto your head. This light is a color of your choosing, a color that you associate with healing. Imagine that this light comes in through the top of your head as you are breathing and then travels throughout your body, vibrating into every cell, every fiber of your body: from the top of your head all the way down your shoulders, into your chest and stomach, into your legs and arms, into your feet and hands. Simply continue to experience this for a little while, perhaps a minute or two. Comfortably hold in mind your intention while doing this.

5. Now unlock your fingers, arms, and legs and set your feet flat on the floor, placing your fingertips in a prayer-like position, the fingertips of the left hand touching the fingertips of your right hand. The palms are not touching. While you hold this position, continue to position the tip of your tongue at the roof of your mouth and to breathe slowly and steadily. Continue to imagine the perpetual light glowing throughout your body. As you are breathing, continue to imagine and feel the breath inhaling and exhaling through the bottom of your feet. Maintain this position for perhaps a minute or two. Comfortably hold in mind your intention for doing this process.

6. Now discontinue this position and notice how you feel. Next place the index and middle fingers of one hand on your forehead between your eyebrows, just your fingers, with light pressure. Take in a deep breath from your diaphragm and then slowly exhale. If you are experiencing any tension or discomfort of any kind, imagine or think that the discomfort is dissipating. You might also think or verbalize this phrase: "Any remaining discomfort is leaving my whole being (or *my body, mind, and soul*)."

7. Now place two fingers under your nose while thinking or announcing, "Any remaining discomfort is leaving my whole being (or *my body, mind, and soul*)." Take a slow deep diaphragmatic breath in and slowly exhale.

8. Next place two fingers under your bottom lip and take a diaphragmatic breath in and slowly exhale while thinking or verbalizing, "Any remaining discomfort is leaving my whole being (or *my body, mind, and soul*)."

9. Next place the fingertips of one hand at the upper section of your chest and take a diaphragmatic breath in and slowly exhale while thinking or verbalizing, "Any remaining discomfort is leaving my whole

being (or *my body, mind, and soul*)." It may help to slowly tap on this section of your chest. Exhale and relax.

10.   Finally, return your awareness to your surroundings and give yourself some time to reorient. Reconsider the issue for which you intended HELP. In most instances the symptom will be relieved or will no longer carry a negative emotional charge. The process may need to be repeated a few times for you to realize substantial benefit. It should be noted that the process is often best considered to be part of a comprehensive treatment approach. Your therapist will likely include other treatments during your therapy sessions.

Chapter 8

TEST AND TREATMENT
POINTS CATALOG

A picture is worth a thousand words.

PSYCHOLOGICAL DISTURBANCES are maintained simultaneously at many levels of functioning. These include activity related to cognition, musculature, brain anatomy, neurochemistry, hormones, cellular components such as cytoskeleton and microtubules, and subtle energies. It appears that some conditions are treated more effectively at one level than another, although one would assume that treatment directed at a primary level would generally alleviate disturbance manifested at secondary or tertiary levels as well. Therefore, treatment applied to the energetic causes will often concurrently resolve chemical and cognitive aspects, unless significant neuroanatomical damage or exogenous factors are involved.

This chapter specifies the various acupoints employed in the diagnosis and treatment of the bioenergy aspects of psychological disturbances.[1] Descriptions and pictures assist the reader in precisely locating the *alarm* or *test* points used to diagnose meridian imbalance (see Figures 6.2a and 6.2b, pp. 104, 105) for illustrations of all 14 alarm or test points), as well as preferred *treatment* points used to further evaluate and alleviate imbalance within the energy system.

---

[1] While the focus of this text is on the application of protocols to address psychological problems, these tools may be useful in diagnosing and treating energy features involved in physical conditions as well.

The reader is advised to become intimately familiar with these diagnostic and treatment points, using this chapter as a manual while actually locating the points on the physical body. This is essential to being able to conduct the diagnostic and treatment protocols that follow.

The practitioner will need to develop skill at therapy localizing these points, each in its own way, in order to discern information about energetic disturbances. Frequently, the subject will be able to touch the point while the examiner checks the indicator muscle. At other times the location of the point is such that it is virtually impossible for the subject to touch it, and therefore this task, with the subject's permission, becomes the responsibility of the examiner. In each instance the examiner must be alert to any confounding effects of the subject's posture with regard to securing accurate information.

Each section of this chapter is arranged by meridians that are categorized according to the location of the respective alarm points used to diagnose meridian imbalance (i.e., six bilateral and six midline meridians). Since it appears that bilateral meridians are somewhat more involved with the right hemisphere and midline meridians are somewhat more left hemispheric, this distinction is also noted. This distinction makes it possible for the examiner to utilize the *hemisphere dominance test* (HDT) to efficiently locate the meridian or meridians involved in the disturbance. It should be noted that sometimes both hemispheres will test weak when one conducts the HDT, and this likely indicates that both hemispheres, and therefore both bilateral and midline meridians, are disrupted at the time that the test is being conducted.[2] While this presents a problem in terms of using the HDT to choose one meridian at a time, it may expand the model to treat a wider range of patients with more complex conditions. At such times, a *single-point protocol* may not be advisable and we may turn to a *multi-point protocol* instead (see Chapter 9).

Each section on a specific meridian begins by locating the alarm point, which is initially used to diagnose or locate the general area of disruption within the energy system. Affirmations that have been used to restore balance within the meridian as a whole are also listed (adapted from Diamond, 1985). Several specific treatment points are further therapy localized to more

---

[2] Preliminary clinical tests between the HDT and goggles designed to assess hemisphere dominance support this conclusion. See *Of Two Minds: The Revolutionary Science of Dual Brain Psychology* by Fredric Schiffer (1998).

precisely define the disruption along the meridian.[3] Each point is described according to the standard acupoint numbers, a descriptive term (e.g., *thumb, thumb pad, under eye, under arm,* etc.), the Chinese term, approximate English translation, and some of the uses of the point in acupuncture. Meridians and their abbreviations are listed in accordance with the *Standard International Nomenclature.* For example, *pericardium* is used rather than *circulation sex* and abbreviated as *PC.* Other preferred terms include *triple energizer (TE)* rather than *triple warmer* or *triple heater, LR* rather than *Lv* or *LIV* as abbreviations for the *liver meridian,* etc.

DIAGNOSTIC AND TREATMENT POINTS: BILATERAL MERIDIANS (RIGHT HEMISPHERE)

Lung

The lung meridian has a total of 11 points, extending from the shoulder to the thumb. In this system the three standard points used to treat the lung meridian are LU-9, LU-10, and LU-11 (see Figure 8.1). The alarm point is LU-1. This meridian may be involved in emotional states such as approval-seeking, contempt, depression, disdain, grief, haughtiness, hopelessness, in-

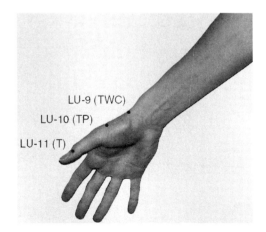

Figure 8.1 Lung meridian diagnostic and treatment points

---

[3]This localization along the meridian is not limited to a physical location, but is believed to represent a specific frequency or energy activity.

tolerance, loneliness, self-pity, prejudice, and scorn. An associated affirmation is *I am humble, tolerant, and modest.*

ALARM POINT: LU-1

The alarm point for the lung meridian is located in a depression one inch below the collarbone on the lateral superior part of the chest in the first intercostal space, approximately six inches from the midline of the sternum near the shoulder. It is called *Chung Fu* or *Mansion of the Center.*

LU-9 THUMB WRIST CREASE (TWC)

This point is located on the palmer side of the skin crease of the wrist, near the hollow created by two tendons in that vicinity. These tendons are attached to the flexor carpi and abductor pollicis longus muscles. This point is referred to as *T'ai Yuan* or *Great Abyss.* In acupuncture it used to treat colds, tonsillitis, malaria, wrist joint and surrounding tissue disease, diabetes mellitus, and deafness.

LU-10 THUMB PAD (TP)

This point is located at the midpoint of the palmer side of the thumb pad, one inch away from the LU-9 or the TWC point. It is referred to as *Yu Chi* or *Fish Border.* In acupuncture this point is needled to treat fever, chills, sore throat, cough, bronchitis, pneumonia, tuberculosis, asthma, dizziness, abdominal pain, back pain, and chest pain.

LU-11 THUMB (T)

This point is located on the radial or outside section of the thumb, the corner where the nail meets the cuticle. It is referred to as *Shao Shang* or *Young Merchant.* In acupuncture this point is used to treat fever, sore throat, tonsillitis, mumps, jaundice, asthma, colds, cough, pneumonia, cerebrovascular disease, coma, indigestion, and psychosis.

Liver

The liver meridian has a total of 14 points, extending from the big toe to below the breast. Four standard points used to treat the liver meridian are LR-3, LR-5, LR-8, and LR-14 (see Figure 8.2). LR-14 is also the alarm point. These points may be involved in emotional states such as anger, aggression, and unhappiness. An associated affirmation is *I am happy and cheerful.*

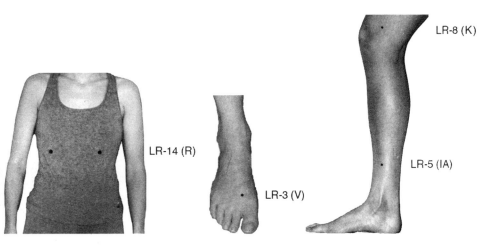

Figure 8.2 Liver meridian diagnostic and treatment points

ALARM POINT: LR-14 RIB (R)

The alarm point for the liver meridian is located on the liver meridian on the mid-clavicular line at the upper edge of the seventh rib at the sixth intercostal space (below the nipple on a male). It is referred to as *Ch'I Men* or *Gate of Hope*. In acupuncture it is used to treat cirrhosis of the liver, angina, urinary retention, enuresis, and hepatitis. Besides being the alarm point for the liver meridian, LR-14 can also be used as a treatment point.

LR-3 VALLEY (V)

This point is located on the dorsal side or top of the foot, in the depression two inches above the webbing between the big and second toes. It is referred to as *T'ai Ch'ung* or *Great Thrust*. In acupuncture it is used to treat headache, dizziness, hernia, pleurisy, and pain in the lower extremities.

LR-5 INSIDE ANKLE (IA)

This point is located five inches above the protrusion of the medial malleolus or innermost ankle bone. It is referred to as *Li Kou* or *Termite Ditch*. In acupuncture it is used to treat impotence, premature ejaculation, and dysmenorrhea.

LR-8 INSIDE OF KNEE (IK)

This point is located on the medial or inside surface of the knee, in the depression where the crease ends when the knee is bent, between the medial epicondyle of the fermur and the semimembranosus tendon. It is referred to as *Ch'u Ch'uan, Fountain of the Bend* or *Crooked Spring*. In acupuncture it is needled to treat dysentery, cirrhosis of the liver, prostate inflammation, irregular menses, prolapsed uterus, knee-joint pain, hemorrhoids, pelvic pain, hysteria, and schizophrenia.

Gallbladder

The gallbladder meridian has a total of 44 points, extending from the bony orbit at the side of the eye to the fourth toe. The four standard points used to treat the gallbladder meridian are GB-1, GB-2, GB-14 (see Figure 8.3), and GB-24. GB-24 is also the alarm point. These points may be involved in emotional states of rage and aggression. An associated affirmation is *I reach out with forgiveness and love.*

ALARM POINT: GB-24 LOWER RIB (LR)

The alarm point for the gallbladder meridian is located on the gallbladder meridian down from the middle of the clavicle below the nipple in the seventh intercostal space, about two inches below the liver alarm point. It is called *Uhr Yueh* or *Sun and Moon*. In acupuncture it is used to treat hepatitis, gastritis, and intercostal neuralgia. Besides being the alarm point for the gallbladder meridian, GB-24 can also be used as a treatment point.

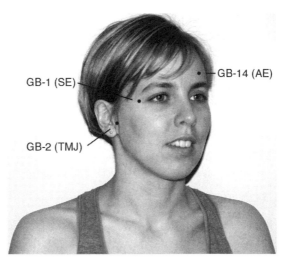

Figure 8.3 Gallbladder meridian diagnostic and treatment points

GB-1 SIDE OF EYE (SE)

This point is located on the temple side of the eye on the bony orbit. Technically it is one-half inch lateral to the lateral ocular angle. It is referred to as *T'ung Tsu Liao* or *Orbit Bone*. In acupuncture it is used to treat headache, night blindness, optic-nerve atrophy, glaucoma, myopia, optic neuritis, facial palsy, and trigeminal neuralgia.

GB-2 TEMPROMANDIBULAR JOINT (TMJ)

When the mouth is open, this point is located in the depression slightly anterior to or in front of and posterior to or below the border of the tragus. It is referred to as *T'ing Hui* or *Hearing Assembly*. In acupuncture it is used to treat deafness, tinnitus, auditory hallucinations, toothache, mumps, and facial palsy.

GB-14 ABOVE EYE (AE)

This point is located one inch above the middle of the eyebrow in the supraorbital notch directly above the pupil when the eyes are directed foreword. It is called *Yang Pai* or *Yang White*. In acupuncture is used to treat night blindness, supraorbital palsy, facial palsy, myopia, and eye disease.

Spleen

The spleen meridian has a total of 21 points, extending from the big toe to approximately six inches beneath the armpit. Three standard points used to treat the spleen/pancreas meridian are SP-1, SP-20, and SP-21 (see Figure 8.4). The alarm point is LR-13 on the liver meridian. These points may be

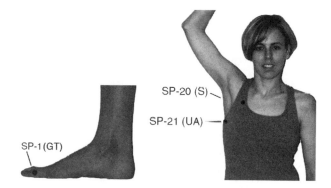

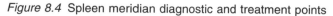

Figure 8.4 Spleen meridian diagnostic and treatment points

involved in addiction, anxiety, hopelessness, obsession, phobias, shyness, low self-confidence, low self-esteem, timidity, and worry. An associated affirmation is *I have faith and confidence in my future*.

ALARM POINT: LR-13

The alarm point for the spleen meridian is located on the liver meridian at the lower end of the tip of the eleventh rib, in the vicinity of the side of the waist. It is referred to as *Chang Men* or *Chapter Gate*. In acupuncture it is used to treat hepatitis, cirrhosis of the liver, vomiting, pleurisy, abdominal distention, and bronchial asthma.

SP-1 GREAT TOE (GT)

This point is located on the medial side of the big toe, slightly out from the nail. It is referred to as *Yin Pai* or *Hidden White*. In acupuncture it is used to treat coma, peritonitis, acute gastroenteritis, dysmenorrhea, gastrointestinal bleeding, and schizophrenia.

SP-20 SHOULDER (S)

This point is located in the space between the second and third ribs, six inches away from the center of the chest bone and in the direction of the shoulder. It is referred to as *Chou Jung* or *Encircling Glory*. In acupuncture it is used to regulate the function of the stomach, to relieve cough and asthma.

SP-21 UNDER ARM (UA)

This point is located on the mid-axillary line about six inches under the armpit, when the arm is raised. It is referred to as *Ta Pao* or *Great Enveloping*. In acupuncture it is used to treat pain in the chest, asthma, whole-body pain, weakness of the extremities, bronchitis, rheumatoid arthritis, pieuritus, pleurisy, and pericarditis.

Kidney

The kidney meridian has a total of 27 points, extending from the plantar surface of the foot to the collarbone next to the sternum. Three standard points used to treat the kidney meridian are K-1, K-3, and K-27 (see Figure 8.5). These points may be involved in addictive urges, anxiety, indecision, phobias, and sexual insecurity. An associated affirmation is *I am sexually secure*.

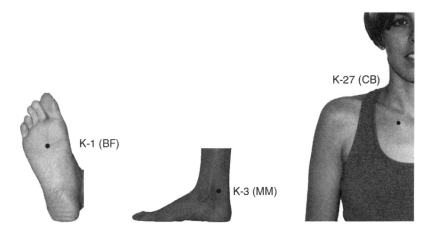

Figure 8.5 Kidney meridian diagnostic and treatment points

ALARM POINT: GB-25

The alarm point for the kidney meridian is located on the gallbladder meridian in the side lumbar region on the lower portion of the front tip of the twelfth floating rib. It is called *Ching Men* or *Gate of Capitol*. In acupuncture it is used to treat diarrhea, vomiting, abdominal distention, lumbar pain, and facial edema.

K-1 BOTTOM OF FOOT (BF)

This point is located approximately one-third of the distance between the base of the toes and the heel of the foot, in the crease on the sole between the second and third toes. It is referred to as *Yung Chuan* or *Bubbling Spring*. In acupuncture it is used to treat headache, shock, heat stroke, hoarseness of the voice, sore throat, cough, acute tonsillitis, tachycardia, jaundice, prolapse of the uterus, spasm of the lower extremities, hernia, edema, and impotence.

K-3 MEDIAL MALLEOLUS (MM)

This point is located in the hollow at the posterior or upper back border of the medial malleolus or innermost ankle bone on the big toe side of the foot. It is between the posterior border of the medial malleolus and the anterior border of the tendon calcaneus. It is referred to as *T'ai Chi* or *Bigger Stream*. In acupuncture it is needled for nephritis, cystitis, dysmenorrhea, toothache, throat inflammation, dizziness, emphysema, hypochondriasis, lower-back pain, and paralysis of the lower extremities.

K-27 COLLARBONE (CB)

This point is located directly under the clavicle or collarbone, in a hollow next to the sternum or chest bone. It is called *Yu Fu* or *Home of Associated Points*. In acupuncture it is used to treat cough, chest pain, bronchitis, bronchial asthma, pleuritis, pleurisy, and neurogenic vomiting.

Large Intestine

The large intestine meridian has a total of 20 points, extending from the tip of the index finger to the side of the nose. Three standard points used to treat the large intestine meridian are LI-1, LI-4, and LI-20 (see Figure 8.6). These points may be involved in emotional states such as guilt, grief, low self-worth, and sadness. An associated affirmation is *I am clean and good.*

ALARM POINT: ST-25

The alarm point for the large intestine meridian is located on the stomach meridian two inches lateral to and two-thirds of an inch below the navel. It is called *T'ien Ch'u* or *Heavenly Pivot*. In acupuncture it is used to treat dysentery, diarrhea, appendicitis, abdominal distention, constipation, and irregular menses.

LI-1 INDEX FINGER (IF)

This point is located on the radial side of the index finger (next to the thumb), on the corner where the nail meets the cuticle. It is referred to as *Shang Yang* or *Consultant Yang*. In acupuncture these points are used to treat fever, glaucoma, deafness, dizziness, toothache, shoulder pain, and tonsillitis, and to reduce swelling in the jaw and throat.

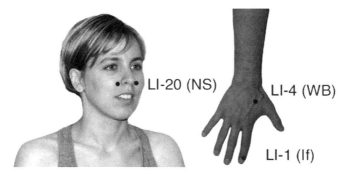

LI-20 (NS)

LI-4 (WB)

LI-1 (If)

Figure 8.6 Large intestine meridian diagnostic and treatment points

LI-4 WEBBING (WB)

This point is located on the dorsal side or back of the hand between the thumb and index fingers, at the midpoint of the radial margin of the second metacarpal (index finger) bone — at the highest part of the first and second metacarpal muscles when the thumb and index finger are adducted. It is referred to as *Ho Ku* or *Joining the Valley*. In acupuncture this point is used to treat fever, colds, pain, facial palsy and spasm, hemiplegia, constipation, sweating, mumps, hysteria, neurosis, and schizophrenia, and to tranquilize the mind to stop convulsions.

LI-20 NASAL SULCUS (NS)

This point is located one-half inch lateral to the nasolabial groove or indentation on the side of the nostril. It is referred to as *Ying Hsiang* or *Welcome Fragrance*. In acupuncture this point is used to treat fever, sinusitis, nasal polyps, facial palsy, and constipation.

MIDLINE MERIDIANS (LEFT HEMISPHERE)

Pericardium

The pericardium meridian has a total of nine points, extending from the vicinity of the nipple to the inside tip of the middle fingernail. Four standard points used to treat the pericardium meridian are PC-6, PC-7, PC-8, and PC-9 (see Figure 8.7). These points may be involved in addiction, anxiety, jealousy, overexcitement, phobias, regret, sexual tension, and stubbornness. An associated affirmation is *I am generous and relaxed*.

ALARM POINT: CV-17

The alarm point for the pericardium meridian is located on the central vessel two inches above the lower tip of the xiphoid process. On men it can be located at the midpoint of the sternum between the nipples. On women it can be located at the level of the fourth intercostal space. It is called *Hsien Chung* or *Center of Altar*. In acupuncture it is used to treat pneumonia, angina, coma, bronchitis, bronchial asthma, and chest pain.

PC-6 WRIST (W)

This point is located at the middle of the palmer side of the forearm, two inches above the transverse wrist crease, between the tendons of the flexor carpi radialis and the palmaris longus muscles. It is referred to as *Nei Kuan*

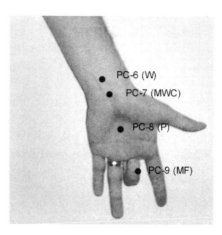

Figure 8.7 Pericardium meridian diagnostic and treatment points

or *Inner Gate*. In acupuncture this point is used to treat motion sickness, tachycardia, rheumatic heart disease, pericarditis, angina pectoris, chest pain, stomach and abdominal pain, headache, hyperthyroidism, epilepsy, hysteria, asthma, throat pain, and hand pain.

PC-7 MIDDLE WRIST CREASE (MWC)

This point is located on the palmer side of the transverse wrist crease between the center and radial or thumb-side tendons (i.e., tendons of the flexor carpi radialis and palmaris longus muscles). It is referred to as *Ta Ling* or *Big Mound*. In acupuncture it is needled for myocarditis, tachycardia, angina pectoris, gastritis, tonsillitis, insomnia, headache, pleurisy, convulsions, shock, and schizophrenia.

PC-8 PALM (P)

This point is located at the proximal transverse or center skin crease of the palm, between the second and third metacarpals, and close to the lateral side of the third metacarpal. It is referred to as *Lao Kung* or *Palace of Labor*. In acupuncture it is used to treat angina, hysteria, psychosis, finger numbness, sweating, stroke, nausea, and hemorrhoids.

PC-9 MIDDLE FINGER (MF)

This point is located on the radial nail side (i.e., next to the index finger) of the middle finger, where the nail meets the cuticle on the side of the finger. It is called *Chung Ch'ung* or *Central Thrust*. In acupuncture it is needled for headache, sore throat, fever, shoulder pain, and nausea.

Heart

The heart meridian has a total of nine points, extending from the armpit to the inside tip of the little fingernail. Four standard points used to treat the lung meridian are HT-3, HT-7, HT-8, and HT-9 (see Figure 8.8). These points may be involved in anger, guilt, hostility, insecurity, overexcitement, sadness, and inability to trust. An associated affirmation is *I have forgiveness in my heart.*

ALARM POINT: CV-14

The alarm point for the heart meridian is located on the central vessel on the mid abdominal line one inch below the tip of the xiphoid process and six inches above the navel. It is called *Chu Ch'ueh* or *Great Shrine.* In

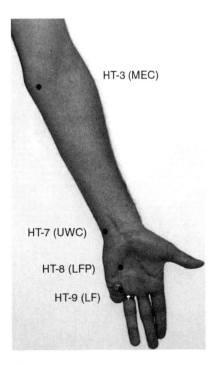

Figure 8.8 Heart meridian diagnostic and treatment points

acupuncture it is used to treat cough, abdominal distention, convulsions, syncope, and schizophrenia.

HT-3 MEDIAL ELBOW CREASE (MEC)

This point is located on the ulnar or inside skin crease of the elbow (toward the torso), at the midpoint between the medial epicondyle of the humerus and the ulnar side of the tendon of the biceps brachialis muscle. This point is located by bending the elbow forward and noting the crease on the torso side of the arm, where the crease ends. It is referred to as *Shao Hai* or *Lesser Sea*. In acupuncture these points are used to promote blood circulation, to relieve mental stress, and to treat headache, epilepsy, angina, pectoris, pleurisy, caries, toothache, dizziness, and tuberculosis.

HT-7 ULNAR WRIST CREASE (UWC)

This point is located on the little finger side of the wrist crease, in the depression of the lateral side of the tendon of the flexor carpi ulnaris muscle. It is referred to as *Shen Men* or *Spirit Gate*. In acupuncture it is used to treat fevers, tachycardia, insomnia, angina, pectoris, convulsions, tongue numbness, nightmares, hysteria, neuroses, and psychoses, and generally to reduce anxiety.

HT-8 LITTLE FINGER PALM (LFP)

When the hand is clenched, this point is located on the middle crease of the palm, between the little and ring fingers. It is referred to as *Shao Fu* or *Lesser Mansion*. In acupuncture it is used to treat hysteria, neuroses, chronic tonsillitis, angina, pectoris, tachycardia, chest pain, arm and forearm numbness, fever, and arthritis of the elbow and wrist.

HT-9 LITTLE FINGER (LF)

This point is located on the radial or inside tip of the little finger, where the nail meets the cuticle. It is referred to as *Shao Ch'Ung* or *Lesser Thrust*. In acupuncture it is used to treat mental stress, tachycardia, angina, pectoris, myocarditis, hepatitis, jaundice, hysteria, epilepsy, shock, and schizophrenia.

Stomach

The stomach meridian has a total of 45 points, extending from directly under the eye to the second toe. Four standard points used to treat the stomach meridian are ST-1, ST-4, ST-12, and ST-45 (see Figure 8.9). These points

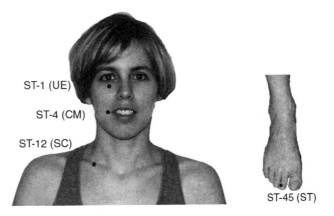

Figure 8.9 Stomach meridian diagnostic and treatment points

may be involved in addiction, anxiety, bitterness, deprivation, despair, disappointment, disgust, greed, phobias, restlessness, and tension. An associated affirmation is *I am content and tranquil.*

ALARM POINT: CV-12

The alarm point for the stomach meridian is located on the central vessel on the mid abdominal line midway between the xiphoid process and the navel. It is called *Chung Kuan* or *Middle Channel.* In acupuncture it is used to treat stomach pain, abdominal distention, nausea, diarrhea, indigestion, vomiting, convulsions, hypertension, bronchial asthma, hysteria, and schizophrenia.

ST-1 UNDER EYE (UE)

With the eyes directed forward, this point is located at the midpoint of the bony orbit under the pupil. It is referred to as *Ch'eng Ch'i* or *Receive Tears.* In acupuncture the two UE points are used to improve visual acuity and to treat myopia and optic nerve atrophy.

ST-4 CORNER OF MOUTH (CM)

This point is located slightly out from the corner of the mouth, 0.4 inch lateral to the oral angle. It is referred to as *Ti Ts'ang* or *Storehouse of Earth.* In acupuncture the CM points are used to treat facial palsy, cerebrovascular disease, toothache, mouth ulcer, and excessive salivation. They are also used to tranquilize the mind.

ST-12 SUPRA-CLAVICULAR (SC)

This point is located at the upper section of the middle of the clavicle or collarbone, directly above the nipple on males. It is referred to as *Ch'Ueh P'En* or *Half a Bowl*. In acupuncture the SC points are used to treat disorders of the diaphragm, cough, asthma, shoulder pain, and tuberculosis.

ST-45 SECOND TOE (ST)

This point is located on the nail of the second toe, on the side away from the big toe. It is on the lateral side of the second toe, one-tenth of an inch lateral and proximal to the nail root. It is referred to as *Li Tui* or *General Exchange*. In acupuncture it is used to treat syncope, fever, facial edema, facial palsy, toothache, abdominal distention, convulsions, hysteria, tonsillitis, anemia, and hepatitis.

Triple Energizer

The triple energizer meridian has a total of 23 points, extending from the ring finger to the outer edge of the eyebrow. Three standard points used to treat the triple energizer meridian are TE-1, TE-3, and TE-23 (see Figure 8.10). These points may be involved in emotional states of depression, deprivation, despair, emptiness, grief, hopelessness, and loneliness. An associated affirmation is *I am light and buoyant*.

ALARM POINT: CV-5

The alarm point for the triple energizer meridian is located on the central vessel on the mid abdominal line one and a half inches below the navel.

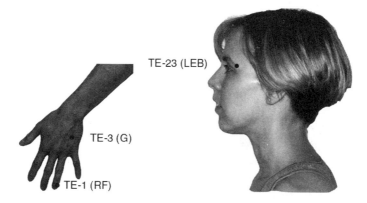

TE-23 (LEB)

TE-3 (G)

TE-1 (RF)

Figure 8.10 Triple energizer meridian diagnostic and treatment points

It is called *Shimen* or *Gate of Stone*. In acupuncture it is used to treat abdominal pain, hernia, urinary tract obstruction, edema, and dysentery.

TE-1 RING FINGER (RF)

This point is located on the ulnar side of the ring fingernail, the side that faces the little finger. It is referred to as *Kuan Ch'ung* or *Passageway for Thrust*. In acupuncture it is used to treat headache, sore throat, fever, shoulder pain, and nausea.

TE-3 GAMUT SPOT (G)

This point is located on the dorsal side or back surface of the hand, between and approximately one inch above the little and ring finger knuckles (in the direction of the wrist). It is referred to as *Chung Chu* or *Central Islet*. In acupuncture it is needled for deafness, tinnitus, headache, colds, shoulder pain, pleurisy, sore throat, and fever.

TE-23 LATERAL EDGE OF EYEBROW (LEB)

This point is located on the lateral or temple side of the eyebrow. It is referred to as *Szu Chu K'ung* or *Silk Bamboo Hollow*. In acupuncture it is used to treat headache, eye problems, facial palsy, convulsion, and schizophrenia.

Small Intestine

The small intestine meridian has a total of 19 points, extending from the outside tip of the little fingernail to the tragus. Three standard points used to treat the small intestine meridian are SI-1, SI-3, and SI-4 (see Figure 8.11). These points may be involved in emotional states such as feelings of

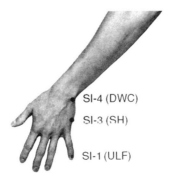

Figure 8.11 Small intestine meridian diagnostic and treatment points

abandonment, overexcitement, irritability, sadness, and shyness. An associated affirmation is *I am full of joy.*

ALARM POINT: CV-4

The alarm point for the small intestine meridian is located on the central vessel on the mid abdominal line three inches below the navel and two inches above the superior border of symphysis pubis. It is called *Kuan Yuan* or *Point of Original Chi.* In acupuncture it is used to treat enuresis, urine retention, impotence, premature ejaculation, nocturnal emission, dysmenorrhea, female infertility, irregular menses, pelvic inflammatory disease, and urinary tract inflammation.

SI-1 ULNAR LITTLE FINGER (ULF)

This point is located on the ulnar or outside tip of the little finger, where the nail meets the cuticle, about one-tenth of an inch lateral and inferior to the nail root. It is referred to as *Shao Chih* or *Lesser Marsh.* In acupuncture it is indicated to treat headache, mumps, insufficient milk, hepatitis, coma, cerebrovascular disease, convulsions, and pleurisy.

SI-3 SIDE OF HAND (SH)

This point is located on the medial edge of the palm or little finger side of the hand, where the palm crease closest to the fingers meets the side of the hand, when the hand is half clenched. It is referred to as *Hou Ch'i* or *Back Stream.* In acupuncture it is used to treat malaria, epilepsy, psychoses, hysteria, pleurisy, cold sweats, neck strain, deafness, back pain, and tonsillitis.

SI-4 DORSAL WRIST CREASE (DWC)

This point is located on the medial or little finger side of the palm in the depression back of the hand near the wrist, between the base of the fifth metacarpal and the pisiform bone. It is at the dorsal wrist crease on the ulnar side. This point is referred to as *Wan Ku* or *Wrist Bone.* In acupuncture it is used to treat fever, headache, common cold, neck stiffness, jaundice, wrist weakness, pleurisy, vomiting, diabetes mellitus, hepatitis, hysteria, and schizophrenia.

Bladder

The bladder meridian has a total of 67 points, extending from the inside edge of the eye to the outside tip of the little toenail. Three standard points used to treat the bladder meridian are BL-1, BL-2, and BL-10 (see Figure 8.12). These points may be involved in frustration, impatience, restlessness, timidity, and trauma. An associated affirmation is *I am at peace*.

ALARM POINT: CV-3

The alarm point for the bladder meridian is located on the central vessel on the mid abdominal line four inches below the navel and on the pubic bone. It is called *Chung Chi* or *Central Pole*. In acupuncture it is used to treat enuresis, urine retention, impotence, premature ejaculation, nocturnal emission, irregular menses, female infertility, sciatic pain, and pelvic inflammatory disease.

BL-1 UNDER EYEBROW (UEB)

This point is located beneath the inside edge of the eyebrow in the hollow next to the eye, above the tear ducts. It is called *Ching Ming* or *Eyes Bright*. In acupuncture this point is used to improve visual acuity.

BL-2 EYEBROW (EB)

This point is located at the medial or inside end of the eyebrow near the bridge of the nose. It is referred to as *T'zan Chu* or *Drilling Bamboo*. In acupuncture this point is used to reduce fever and improve visual acuity. Other clinical indications include headache, glaucoma, excessive tearing, myopia, and nystagmus.

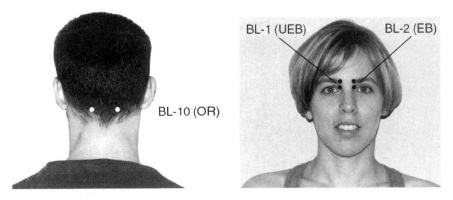

Figure 8.12 Bladder meridian diagnostic and treatment points

BL-10 OCCIPITAL RIDGE (OR)

This point is located below and on the side of the occipital ridge at the back of the head, on the ropy muscles, one and a third inches lateral to the posterior midline in the superior margin of the spinous process of the axis. It is referred to as *Tien Chu* or *Heavenly Pillar*. In acupuncture it is used to treat fever, headache, stiff neck, sore throat, hysteria, convulsions, schizophrenia, hypochondriasis, common cold, and insomnia.

COLLECTOR MERIDIANS

There are eight extraordinary vessels in the meridian system. The best known are the *conception* or *central vessel*, which extends the midline at the front of the body, and the *governing vessel*, which begins under the upper lip and extends down the midline at the back of the body. These meridians are neither bilateral nor midline meridians. They cannot be evaluated via the HDT.

Conception Vessel

The conception vessel has a total of 24 points, extending from the center of the perineum to the depression between the chin and lower lip. Two standard points used to treat the conception vessel are CV-22 and CV-24 (see Figure 8.13). These points may be involved in feelings of shame. An associated affirmation is *I am worthy*.

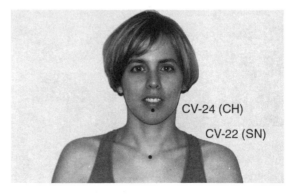

Figure 8.13 Conception vessel diagnostic and treatment points

TEST POINT: CV-24 CHIN (CH)[4]

The test point for the central vessel is located on the central vessel in the depression between the lower lip and the chin. It is called *Ch'eng Chiang* or *Receiving Fluid*. In acupuncture it is used to treat excessive salivation, toothache, facial palsy, mouth ulcer, and cerebrovascular disease.

CV-22 SUPERSTERNAL NOTCH (SN)

This point is located one-half inch above the middle of the hollow at the superior or upper margin of the jugular notch of the sternum, in the hollow below the Adam's apple. It is referred to as *T'ien T'u* or *Heaven Rushing*.

Governing Vessel

The governing vessel has a total of 28 points, extending from the tip of the coccyx to the junction between the frenulum of the upper lip and gingiva. Three standard points used to treat the governing vessel are GV-17, GV-24.5, and GV-26 (see Figure 8.14). These points may be involved in feelings of embarrassment. An associated affirmation is *I am at ease.*

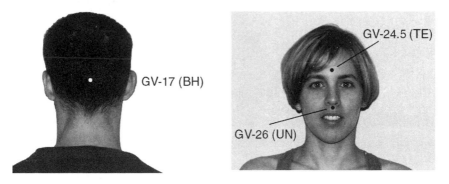

Figure 8.14 Governing vessel diagnostic and treatment points

---

[4]The central vessel does not have an alarm point. CV-24 is used as the test point.

TEST POINT: GV-26 UNDER NOSE (UN)[5]

The test point for the governing vessel is located on the governing vessel in the depression below the nose at junction of philtrum and upper lip in the upper third of the nasolabial groove. It is called *Shui Kou* or *Ditch*. In acupuncture it is used to treat shock, car and sea sickness, coma, heat stroke, convulsions, and hysteria.

GV-17 BACK OF HEAD (BH)

This point is located on the mid sagittal line at the back of the head, above the external occipital protuberance. It is referred to as *Nao Hu* or *Shelter of the Brain*. In acupuncture it is used to treat dizziness, neck stiffness, hypertension, epilepsy, hysteria, and jaundice.

GV-24.5 THIRD EYE (TE)

This point is located between the eyebrows at the indentation where the nose meets the forehead. It is not a specific acupoint; rather it is located midway between GV-24 on the upper section of the forehead and GV-25 on the tip of the nose. Known by various names, such as *Ajna Chakra*, *Spiritual Eye*, and *Third Eye*, it is, according to the Hindus, the major nerve center in the human body. Hindus wear a tilak, a sandalwood paste red dot for women and an elongated dot for men, at this location as a reminder of wedding vows and to cool the nerve center associated with this location. It is said to calm and quiet the mind.

The treatment points described in this chapter were chosen on the basis of their ease of location and effectiveness in balancing the energy system. In addition, out of concern for the relationship between subject and examiner, I have avoided acupoints that are located in areas of the anatomy that are best not attended to in psychotherapy practices for reasons of modesty, as well as various ethical and legal concerns. Excluding points at "questionable" locations does not appear to hinder therapeutic effectiveness, although it is conceivable that at a future time we will learn that some of these excluded points must be touched to help patients with certain conditions.

While more globally focused approaches such as HELP and NAEM (see Chapter 7) are highly effective in treating a variety of problems, with many

---

[5]The governing vessel does not have an alarm point. GV-26 is used as the test point.

complex and chronic problems precision diagnosis and treatment is often necessitated in order to realize positive, ongoing results. This is why the treatment points highlighted in the present chapter are important. The next chapter covers the *single-point* and *multi-point protocols*. These precision diagnostic approaches make it possible to specifically tailor the treatments to the individual.

Chapter 9

SINGLE-POINT AND MULTI-POINT PROTOCOLS

Give me a place to stand and I will move the Earth.

—*Archimedes*

THE SINGLE-POINT PROTOCOL is employed when global treatments, such NAEM and HELP, or when algorithms (Gallo, 1998) do not achieve adequate results. At other times the therapist may prefer to employ this protocol in order to examine the energetic structure of the psychological condition and/or to treat the problem efficiently. The information obtained by this protocol can also provide the client with a highly efficient means of self-treatment for conditions that require ongoing in vivo attention. For example, while a global treatment protocol may be an important component in the comprehensive treatment of depression, generalized anxiety, and self-esteem issues, it is not a viable way of treating a panic attack or phobic reaction in vivo, where the single-point protocol is highly efficient.

The guiding assumption of the single-point protocol is that the energy disruptions at the basis of a psychological problem can be efficiently treated by addressing one acupoint at a time. The protocol entails locating a single treatment point and then having the client physically tap or percuss that point in order to stimulate the energy system and thus remove the negative affects or emotions associated with the psychological problem. Here it is assumed that this point is *principally* involved in the energy disruption. Even though other meridians and associated acupoints may be involved in a condition, treatment of the *nodal point* will efficiently reverberate throughout the energy system and neutralize the problem. Theoretically we assume that there is an affect-perturbation connection and that stimulating the energy system at a specific locale serves to collapse or subsume the perturbations in the thought field germane to the psychological problem.

This procedure involves getting as much effect out of a single point as possible before moving on to another associated acupoint. While a single point will often prove sufficient, the protocol dictates that, if the acupoint has reached its limits and the problem has not been thoroughly alleviated, another high signal strength point be addressed. When additional points need to be addressed, it is likely that each point is associated with a relatively distinct but interrelated energetic aspect of the problem. When this protocol proves effective, rarely will it be necessary to address more than a few points in order to achieve the desired outcome of neutralizing the negative emotional components.

SINGLE-POINT PROTOCOL

Preparation

Prior to conducting the single-point protocol the therapist should address a number of preliminary considerations: building rapport, obtaining an appropriately thorough history, developing a sufficiently comprehensive treatment plan, administering relevant questionnaires and psychometrics when needed, explaining the purpose and method involved in energy diagnostics and treatment, and securing permission to proceed in this manner.

1. Introductory Statement

The introduction of manual muscle testing is covered in Chapter 3. Two scripts for introducing the concept of energy psychology and the method of muscle testing can be found on pages 40–41 and 41–42.

2. Qualifying the Indicator Muscle

Prior to conducting manual muscle testing or checking, the indicator muscle should be qualified. To do this the therapist inquires if the client will let him/her press on the arm while isolating a deltoid muscle (or apply pressure to whatever muscle is chosen). The purpose here is to screen for any contraindications to using that muscle, such as a physical problem.

3. *Preliminary Calibration Tests*

It is useful to begin with a few preliminary tests or demonstrations of the muscle testing phenomenon. The examiner can test *in the clear*, that is, ask the subject to "hold" and then press on the extended arm.[1] This provides a baseline or measure of the subject's ability to hold the muscle firm. After this phase, follow-up challenges can be compared to this baseline.

The subject can then be asked to state his/her name, prefaced by the statement, "My name is *(correct name)*." Checking the indicator muscle should result in a response similar to or firmer than the baseline response. Next the subject can be asked to state a false name, again prefaced by, "My name is *(wrong name)*." This time the indicator muscle response should be relatively weaker. Other preliminary tests can be conducted regarding what the subject ate at a specific meal, identifying the President of the United States, thinking about something pleasant as compared to something unpleasant, etc. In each instance the subject's attention should be directed to observing and understanding the relevance of the muscle response.

4. *Diagnosing and Correcting Neurologic Disorganization/Switching*

If a clear distinction between muscle responses is detectable, the presence of neurologic disorganization is unlikely and the muscle response is adequate for making finer diagnostic determinations. If it is difficult or impossible to distinguish between weak and strong muscle responses, this needs to be investigated further and corrected, as outlined in Chapter 4; otherwise, the single-point protocol cannot be conducted.

5. *Diagnosing and Correcting Massive Psychological Reversal*

Next it is recommended that the examiner determine if massive psychological reversal (MPR) is present. MPR is a reversal across many contexts. This may or may not be relevant in the specific area for which the client is seeking therapy, although massively reversed clients can often benefit from more extensive treatment, even if they are only presenting for a delimited issue

---

[1] For ease of discussion, from this point on the straight arm test (isolating the middle deltoid as the indicator muscle) will be used. I recognize that this will not be the appropriate measure for some subjects.

such as a specific phobia. See Chapter 5 for the diagnosis and treatment of massive psychological reversal.

6. Accessing the Problem State

If the client is not neurologically disorganized, it is possible to detect when the problem is attuned. The examiner asks the subject to think about the problem. It is not necessary to visualize the problem, although some may find this an effective way to attune at a high signal strength level. After the problem is attuned, the subject is asked to hold while the indicator muscle is challenged. In a majority of cases the muscle will not remain firm, thus corroborating that the problem thought field is attuned.

7. Scaling

It is helpful to ask the subject to rate the subjective units of distress (SUD) 0–10, either before or after challenging the indicator muscle while the problem is being attuned. The examiner might ask, "As you think about the problem at this very moment [e.g., phobia, trauma, depression], on a scale of 0–10, with 10 being the highest level of discomfort and 0 being no discomfort at all, how much discomfort do you feel?" After the subject offers a number, the SUD can be further corroborated by challenging the indicator muscle. Although the indicator muscle will usually test weak (off) when problem state is attuned, it will test strong (on) when the SUD rating is stated.

In most cases the SUD and muscular ratings will be equivalent; however, when they do not coincide, the examiner and subject can determine the precise muscular rating by muscle testing. Specifically, the subject states various ratings and the examiner challenges the muscle each time. For example, the subject may state, "It's a 5," after which the examiner checks the muscle. If the muscle remains firm, the rating is accepted as accurate; if the muscle becomes slack, the rating is rejected and another rating is tested. This procedure assists the client and examiner in obtaining an accurate pre-measure upon which to assess progress toward the goal of alleviating the emotional distress.

When the stated SUD and the rating obtained by muscle testing do not agree, the therapist should simply tell the client that, while there is a differ ence, the client is really the world's best authority on how he/she feels. It might also be pointed out that the distinction here is between how the client feels and the energetic structure underlying the feelings. We want to know both the SUD and the muscular units of distress (MUD), since each provides distinct information. For example, if after treatment the client were to report a SUD of 0 and MUD of 6, this would suggest that the problem was still energetically present even though the client was unable to detect its presence. Alternatively, if the SUD were 5 and the MUD were 0, this would suggest that the problem was gone and that the individual would experience the change shortly.

8.   Resonance Locking

Once attuned, the perturbed thought field will usually continue to resonate long enough so that the diagnostic procedure can be completed. This suggests a kind of entrainment or resonance lock, which can be described in terms of a reverberating of the energetic aspects of the problem state or perhaps also in terms of subconscious awareness. No doubt neurologic and chemical components are also involved in the experience. Regardless of how this is conceptualized, we know from experience that when we think about something that is notably disturbing, the feelings associated with the thought continue to linger for a time even after the thought has been consciously dismissed.

Even though resonating is likely, we cannot be assured that the signal strength will remain sufficiently elevated for proper diagnosis of the energetic aspects of the problem. This may be a function of the degree to which the client is able consciously to access the thought field or intervening thought fields. This problem can be overcome by employing a simple resonance locking procedure such as the leg lock (also referred to as pause lock) or the glabella tap, as described on pages 115–118. Both of these procedures promote the locking in of "whole body information" without the client being required to consciously think about and experience distress about the issue being treated. This is also of value when treating potentially highly distressing material, such as traumas, that tend to produce high levels of abreaction or even dissociative episodes.

9.   Diagnosing and Correcting Specific Psychological Reversal

Once the psychological issue is attuned and locked in, the examiner can test for and correct psychological reversals, as described in Chapter 5.

10.   Diagnosing and Correcting Other Reversals

Next the therapist may wish to rule out alternative reversals, including deep level and criteria-related reversals, as described in Chapter 5. Deep level is assessed by having the client state, "I *will* be over this problem" vs. "I *will* continue to have this problem." There are many types of criteria-related reversals, the most common ones relating to deserving ("I *deserve* to get over this problem"), safety ("It's *safe* for me to get over this problem"), and possibility ("It's *possible* for me to get over this problem"). Testing for these levels is usually sufficient, although knowledge about the client will often alert the therapist as to other criteria that may block the resolution of the psychological problem.

After educating clients about the nature of reversals, some examiners screen for them by challenging the indicator muscle to a statement such as, "There is a reversal (or another reversal, or other reversals) blocking the resolution of this problem."

Some therapists have also experimented with all inclusive or universal corrections for psychological reversals once reversal has been diagnosed. The procedures for this correction are described on pages 100–101.

11.   The Hemisphere Dominance Test (HDT)

In many instances the experienced practitioner will be able to accurately intuit which meridians are involved, given the client's presenting complaint. For example, if the issue entails anger, the heart, liver, and gallbladder meridians are likely locations of the energy disruption. When a client refers to guilt or shame, the large intestine and heart meridians, in addition to the central vessel, should be evaluated. However, these are merely possibilities, which need to be diagnosed further via the respective alarm points (see below). Such guesswork can be curtailed by employing the hemisphere dominance test (HDT), which makes it possible quickly to divide the twelve primary meridians by two, thus reducing the number of meridian alarm points to therapy localize.

After the client has attuned the psychological problem and a resonance lock has been established, the therapist directs the client to place the palm of his/her right hand a few inches parallel to and one to three inches from the right side of the head opposite the right ear. At this point the indicator muscle is tested. If the indicator muscle "weakens," the client is right-hemisphere dominant with respect to the problem. If the muscle remains relatively strong, the left hemisphere is tested by having the client place the palm of his/her right hand parallel to and away from the left side of the head opposite the left ear. To do this the client moves his/her right arm and hand across the front of the head and positions the right hand opposite the left ear while the indicator muscle is challenged. If the muscle now tests weak, the subject is said to be left-hemisphere dominant. (See Figure 6.1, p. 103.)

If the *right hemisphere* is revealed to be dominant in the problem state, this indicates an imbalance in at least one of the following *bilateral* meridians: lung, liver, gallbladder, spleen, kidney, large intestine. If the *left hemisphere* is revealed to be dominant in the problem state, this indicates an imbalance in at least one of the following *midline* meridians: pericardium (or circulation-sex), heart, stomach, triple energizer (or triple heater or triple warmer), small intestine, bladder.

A feasible mnemonic device is to observe the position of the client's right elbow during the HDT. When the right hemisphere is being therapy localized, the elbow is on one side, the right side, of the client's body, pointing to one of the bilateral sides, thus indicating bilateral meridians.[2] When the left hemisphere is being therapy localized, the elbow is positioned at the center or midline of the client's torso, thus indicating midline meridians. This device is applicable unless it is necessary to have the client therapy localize the cerebral hemispheres with his/her left palm. In this case the test itself still works, but the mnemonic devise cannot be applied.

Sometimes the indicator muscle tests weak while the examiner therapy localizes *both* right and left hemispheres.[3] Assuming that the muscle test is accurately conducted, this suggests that more than one meridian is simultaneously involved in the structure of the problem and that *both* bilateral and midline meridians are involved. However, in this single-point protocol, it is recommended that the therapist simply accept the first alarm point that tests

---

[2]All of the 12 primary meridians are bilateral, in that there are dual pathways on opposite sides of the body. However, what I am referring to as *bilateral meridians* pertains to *alarm points*, also called *test points*. Each of the midline meridians has only one alarm point along the midline of the body, whereas each of the bilateral meridians has two alarm points, one on each side of the body.

[3]In his original discussion of the test for cerebral dominance, Diamond (1985) did not identify instances of both hemispheres testing weak; however, I have found this to occur in a number of cases.

strong (see following section), rather than attempting to locate all of the meridians involved.[4]

12.   *Therapy Localizing Alarm Points*

The HDT conceivably cuts our work in half. In a broad sense, it zeroes in on six of the twelve primary meridians. At this point it is necessary to further therapy localize within the subset of six meridians via the respective alarm points (see Chapter 8). As directed by the therapist, the client touches each alarm point with the palmar surface of several fingers or the palm of the free hand, while the therapist challenges the indicator muscle.[5] Although therapy localization of alarm points can be done while clothing is covering the areas — natural fibers being preferred in such instances — this can reduce the quality of the test. Although it may not always be practical or permissible, therapy localization is best done by the client touching the skin with his/ her fingers. As a general rule, the therapist should not be the one to touch the alarm points. Aside from the ethical and legal considerations, another person touching the alarm points can also confound the results.

Alarm points can be selected in succession from top to bottom or in accordance with the therapist's informed intuition. Initially, the indicator muscle will be relatively weak, since the psychological problem is in resonance lock. When the alarm point of the principal meridian is challenged, however, the indicator muscle will evidence increased firmness or strength. Essentially, this appears to close a circuit that is disrupted due to the stress of the psychological problem. With the single-point protocol, the therapist stops testing alarm points as soon as a significantly strong muscle response is obtained. While there are times when it is necessary to alternately test two or more meridians in order to determine which one produces the strongest response, the examiner should not get so involved in this process as to fatigue the subject. Excessive muscle testing can confound the results. In most instances first impressions are valid.

While the single-point protocol assumes that it is necessary to address

---

[4]Using the single-point protocol, we do not necessarily assume that there is only one meridian involved in the problem, but rather that it is sufficient to stimulate only one acupoint at a time.

[5]Due to ion balance or possibly neural disorganization, in some instances it will be necessary to have the client therapy localize with the dorsal side of the fingers and hand, since the palmar surface will not yield positive therapy localization (Walther, 1988).

only the principal meridian, it is nonetheless recognized that when an energy disruption occurs it does so in many aspects of the energy system simultaneously. Therefore, there will be instances when additional alarm points will test nearly or even equally as strong. This does not pose a problem from the standpoint of treatment efficacy and effectiveness.

13. Therapy Localizing Treatment Points

When the indicator muscle tests strong while an alarm point is therapy localized, this suggests that there is a disruption in the respective meridian, although it does not reveal precisely where the disruption lies. To consistently follow the principles of therapy localization, further testing along the meridian is needed to find an effective treatment point. Therefore, usually it is not appropriate to lump alarm points and treatment points into the same category. It is also erroneous to assume that there is a one-to-one relationship between alarm points and treatment points, such that each alarm point invariably designates the same meridian treatment point each and every time.

If an energy diagnostic system depends on alarm points for diagnosis, invariably it will be accurate regarding the general location of the energy disruption, since alarm points provide summary information about their respective meridians. However, if only one treatment point is employed for each meridian, there will be instances in which that treatment point will not prove effective in abolishing the energy disruption. In many instances, stimulating the same point will vibrate globally throughout the meridian and treat the meridian as a whole, but this cannot be guaranteed.

If an energy diagnostic system were to abandon alarm points for diagnosis and instead specify therapy localization of a single treatment point for each of the meridians, there would be an increasing number of false negatives. That is, there would be instances in which that specific treatment point would not test positive, suggesting that the meridian was not involved in the problem even though it was. Most treatment points do not offer summary information about the entire meridian in the way that alarm points do.

At this stage of the protocol, the therapist and client therapy localize various treatment points along the involved meridian until a treatment point is localized that again abolishes the muscle weakening.[6] In rare instances

---

[6] Many of the treatment points are difficult for the client to therapy localize. Although it is generally preferred that the client do the touching, most of the treatment points are located in areas where

the examiner discovers that none of the most common points covered in Chapter 8 tests positive, then other points should be explored. For instance, on the pericardium meridian PC-9, PC-8, PC-7, and PC-6 were discussed, even though there are nine pericardium treatment points in all. Therefore, if none of these points tests positive, the therapist has an additional five points to choose from.

14. Stimulating Treatment Points

After an involved treatment point has been localized, the point is stimulated for approximately five to ten seconds. The standard way of doing this is by either the client or therapist tapping on the treatment point with the tips of his/her fingers. Other means of stimulation include simply pressing on or aiming a cold laser beam at the acupoint for several seconds. These approaches may be chosen according to client preferences and particularly when the client experiences physical pain in the acupoint location. The therapist may find added benefit in having the client verbalize several times an affirmation associated with the meridian. For example, if the heart meridian is involved, a possible associated affirmation would be, "I have forgiveness in my heart." If the spleen meridian is involved, the client might say, "I have faith and confidence in my future." Although frequently such affirmations appear to be sufficient for balancing the related aspect of the energy system, it is better to combine the affirmation with physical stimulation of the treatment point.

15. Ongoing Evaluation

Intermittently the therapist may wish to take SUD and MUD readings.[7] As long as the SUD continues to decrease by at least two points with each evaluation, stimulation of the treatment point is resumed until the SUD reaches zero or stops decreasing.

If the SUD rating stops decreasing, the therapist should check for and

---

the therapist can exercise the discretion to therapy localize. However the therapist should also be alert to the possibility that his or her energy level at the time may affect the results, interfering with accurate interpretation.

[7]To reiterate, if a SUD of 5 is reported, the therapist can check further by challenging the indicator muscle after the client says, "I'm now at a 5." If the muscle tests strong, this further corroborates the rating. If the muscle does not hold firm, other ratings are tested. If the SUD and MUD ratings do not coincide, they are rarely off by more than a single point in either direction.

correct any intervening or mini reversal (Callahan, 1985) before continuing stimulation. Possible reversals at this point include the intervening version of specific reversal (i.e., "I want to be *completely* over this problem") or any criteria-related reversal (e.g., deserving, safety, possibility, motivation, deprivation).

If a specific intervening reversal is not revealed, the therapist may choose to check for the common factors that may block treatment progress, trust his/her intuition, or evaluate with a screening statement such as, "There is a reversal (or another reversal, or other reversals) blocking the resolution of this problem." If the presence of an intervening reversal is suggested as a result of testing this statement, the therapist can then explore various options. Again, one should insure that the client has a basic understanding of what a reversal entails. (See Chapter 5 for detailed coverage of reversals.)

16. Balancing Procedures

When the SUD rating has reached zero, or has otherwise stopped decreasing and a reversal is not involved, one of the balancing procedures can be introduced. These include the nine gamut treatments, brain balancing procedure, and cross-crawl exercises. While the therapist can provide one of these procedures in its entirety without bothering to diagnose its necessity, diagnosis provides indications as to which elements of the respective procedure are needed, in addition to verifying that the requirements of the individual elements have been fulfilled. Diagnosis may also reveal that none of these procedures is required. It should be noted that employing these procedures (e.g., specific eye positions, humming, cross-crawl) is also a useful means of assessing and insuring the thoroughness of the treatment effects. (See Chapter 6 for detailed coverage.) In addition, the balancing procedures frequently tune in related energetic aspects of the thought field, making those aspects available for diagnosis and treatment.

17. Reevaluation and Further Treatment

After a balancing procedure has been provided, the therapist once again checks the SUD and MUD ratings. If the ratings are not at zero, and a reversal is not present, the therapist again diagnoses any other meridian imbalance. That is, the HDT → alarm point localization → treatment point localization sequence is repeated. If another treatment point is revealed, it may be within the same or another meridian (i.e., within meridians vs. across meridians). When the next principal meridian treatment point is located, it is stimulated in the same manner as the previous treatment point. This includes physical stimulation, possibly combined with a relevant affirmation, as well as a balancing procedure.

18. Eye Roll Procedures

When the level of discomfort (SUD and MUD) is within 0–2 range, the therapist may introduce either the floor-to-ceiling eye roll (ER) or the elaborated eye roll (EER) in order to reduce the stress level to zero. One of these procedures can simply be provided for "good measure" to be assured that all traces of stress have been removed. (See Chapter 6 for details.)

19. Outcome Projection Procedure

In-session removal of the distress associated with a specific thought field or thought field matrix is frequently all that is needed to alleviate the psychological problem altogether. However, most clients who obtain such immediate and lasting results either have a fairly uncomplicated problem to begin with or possess certain admirable facilities that less fortunate clients lack. When clients have less psychological health and more complex problems, desensitization or collapsing perturbations does not appear to be sufficient. In such situations, failure of the procedure frequently seems to be a function of the therapy not being adequately contextualized. Or it may be related to the results not being incorporated into the client's belief structure.

Contextualization is an age-old psychotherapy issue. Even if the distress is alleviated within the therapeutic setting, this does not guarantee that the results will transfer to the desired context. For example, if a client has a height phobia and is able to experience an elevated SUD while simply thinking about or visualizing looking down from a high ladder, alleviating the thought-induced anxiety may not relieve the anxiety experienced within the real-life setting. While both anxiety responses are fundamentally a function of thought, each is a different kind or quality of thought.

With regard to the client's belief structure concerning the problem, even if the distress is eliminated in the therapy session, real-life transfer may be prevented if the client does not believe that he or she can *really* get over the problem. This may be thought of as a reversal that becomes activated within certain contexts other than the therapy session. The more deeply ingrained the negative belief structure, the more likely that results will degrade within or transfer not at all to the real-life situation.

While there are instances where context and belief structure dictate the need for in vivo treatment, the *outcome projection procedure* can significantly increase the chances of results transfer. This procedure is conducted as follows:

a. The client states the desired outcome (e.g., climb up a 12-foot ladder without anxiety) and then rates how strongly he/she believes that it will occur (0–10, with 10 being the strongest belief level). For example: "At a level X I believe that I will be able to climb a 12-foot ladder without anxiety."

b. The indicator muscle is then tested for corroboration. If the client evidences a belief level of 8–10, this is probably adequate and in most instances results can be expected to transfer easily to the needed context. If the belief level is lower than 8, the therapist guides the client through the diagnostic procedure of locating the involved meridian and treatment point. The first step in this process involves ruling out any specific reversal that could block the transfer of therapeutic results to everyday contexts. Assuming that the belief level is higher than zero, the therapist tests the indicator muscle after directing the client to make a statement such as: "I want to thoroughly believe that I will be able to climb a 12-foot ladder without anxiety" or, "I want my belief level to be an 8 or higher with regard to being able to climb a 12-foot ladder without anxiety." If a reversal is evident, it is corrected in one of the usual ways and then the client is tested again before proceeding. It should be noted that, even if the test indicates that a reversal is not present, a deeper level reversal may be operating; therefore, it may be necessary to evaluate and correct other levels. For example, a deep level reversal may be present, as evidenced by a negative muscle response to the following test statement: "I *will* thoroughly believe that I will be able to climb a 12-foot ladder without anxiety."

c. After reversals have been alleviated, generally there is no indicator muscle weakening when the client attunes "I (*want to, will, etc.,*) thoroughly believe . . ." Nevertheless the client may still report a less-than-desirable belief level, which can be corroborated via muscle testing. At this point the client is directed to tap on triple energizer-3 (gamut spot) or triple energizer-23 while thinking about being able to achieve the desired outcome in context. With repeated application of this aspect of the procedure, the belief level generally elevates into the desired range (i.e., 8–10). The TE-3 or TE-23 tapping can be combined with a balancing procedure and the elaborated eye roll to further enhance results.

d. If indicator muscle weakening is evident after the reversals have been corrected, the therapist may choose to diagnose a treatment point that will efficiently elevate the belief level. This is conducted in the usual way: HDT → alarm point localization → treatment point localization.

e. After the belief level is within the desired range (with or without the outcome projection procedure), the indicator muscle should remain strong and the client should continue to experience a strong belief level while thinking about being in the context in an *associated manner*. That is, the client should be able to create an internal representation (seeing, hearing, feeling) of actually being in the situation without experiencing any indications of distress or of a drop in belief level. The *associated position* is akin to being in the body of the internal image, such that one is able to sense (see, hear, feel) in the same general way as in the actual situation.

f. After the belief level is within the desired range, the indicator muscle should also remain strong while repeating the HDT, which should demonstrate equivalent strength in reference to both hemispheres.

20. *Evidence of Bioenergy Balance*

The indicator muscle generally weakens when a perturbed thought field is attuned. In such instances, therapy localization of an active treatment point results in a strengthening of the indicator muscle. After the treatment point has been thoroughly treated, the muscle should remain strong when the thought field is attuned, assuming that the stress associated with the thought field has been eliminated. After the stress has been alleviated, therapy localization of the point should result in a strong indicator muscle response. If therapy localizing the treatment point results in weakening of the indicator muscle, there is still stress in the system and the treatment point is still active. Therefore, additional treatment directed at that point is needed. Once the thought field is no longer perturbed, the indicator muscle will remain strong with and without therapy localization of the point, and repeating the HDT will reveal a strong indicator muscle while either hemisphere is evaluated.

21. *Validation*

Proving takes place in everyday life. When the results do not hold in everyday life, often other aspects of the problem need to be addressed with this protocol. For example, fear of flying is generally not a singular anxiety, but rather includes anxiety related to take-off, flight turbulence, landing, possibility of crashing, claustrophobia, etc. If the protocol were to alleviate only a couple of these aspects, the problem would not be resolved. Cure would be a function of neutralizing all of the anxieties and also possibly adding some enjoyment in flying.

22. *Assignments*

After the patient has been treated for the problem within the therapy session, it is often beneficial to offer a debriefing and to provide a homework assignment. The patient should be told that symptoms sometimes return due to any variety of factors, including the possibility that not all of the aspects of the problem have been neutralized, increases in psychological stress, substance sensitivities (see Chapter 12), etc. He/she should be provided with instruction (usually written) for repeating the treatment that was found to alleviate the problem during the therapy session. The patient should also be taught how to conduct global treatments such as the NAEM and HELP protocols to cover instances when the individually tailored treatment may not work (see Chapter 7). The therapist should also consider being available for telephone consultation between sessions, since treating symptoms when they emerge increases the overall effectiveness of the therapy. I also choose to teach clients about other methods of dismissing disturbing thought fields, such as through thought awareness. Focused readings are beneficial in this regard.

MULTI-POINT PROTOCOL

The guiding assumption of the multi-point protocol is that the energy disruptions at the basis of a psychological problem can be treated by addressing a cluster of acupoints. The protocol entails locating several simultaneously active treatment points and then having the client physically tap or percuss on those points in order to stimulate the energy system and thus remove the negative affects or emotions associated with the psychological problem. It is assumed that these are the principal meridian points involved in the energy disruption. Theoretically there is assumed to be an affect-perturbation connection and that stimulating the energy system in this more extensive yet precise manner serves to collapse or subsume the perturbations in the thought field specific to the psychological problem.

This procedure involves obtaining as much effect as possible out of a cluster of points before moving on to another associated cluster. While generally a single cluster will prove sufficient, when the original grouping of points has reached its limits and the problem has not been thoroughly alleviated, the protocol dictates that another high signal strength cluster be addressed in order to neutralize the problem. When additional clusters need to be addressed, it is likely that each is associated with a relatively separate significant energetic aspect of the problem.

It should be noted that while the treatment points in a cluster are elicited in a sequence or order, this appears to be merely an artifact of the linear process involved in muscle testing. Obviously only one point at a time can be elicited, even though all of the points in the cluster are simultaneously active. The points need not be treated in the order diagnosed for the problem to be alleviated. Sequential order has little if any relevance in this regard, and considerable clinical experience has confirmed this.

From preparation through therapy localization of treatment points, the multi-point protocol does not differ from the single-point protocol. The reader should be familiar with the first 13 steps of that protocol. We pick up here with step 14.

14. Clear Treatment Point

After a treatment point has been diagnosed, the point is tapped no more than five times to "clear" the meridian, making other relevant meridian points detectable. The tapping is done briefly each time, not with the intention of treating the energy disruption in the way it is done with the single-point protocol, but rather simply to reduce the signal strength of the treatment point so that other high signal strength points will become visible.

15. Repeat Relevant Tests

After the treatment point is briefly stimulated, the same therapy localization process is repeated in order to locate the next relevant treatment point. The recursive process is as follows: HDT → alarm point test → treatment point test → treatment point stimulation. This procedure is repeated until the limit of the cluster is defined, which is evident in a few ways:

a. When the first repetition of a treatment point occurs, this signals the dimensions of the cluster. That is, if the treatment points are *cb* → *cm* → *if* → *or* → *cm*, the limit of the cluster is evident as soon as *cm* occurs for the second time. This is an important consideration, since if we were to look for a sequence instead of a cluster, we would not know to stop testing at this point. Conceivably the treatment points could go on indefinitely.

b. When the indicator muscle tests relatively strong, this is another indication that the cluster has been thoroughly defined.

c. The therapist can test the indicator muscle after having the client say, "This is the limit of the cluster." A strong muscle response indicates that the cluster has been adequately defined.

d. Finally, the therapist can simply stop testing after a maximum of five treatment points has been revealed. In most instances this will prove sufficient, even though some additional distinct points might be revealed with continuation of the diagnostic process. Most likely any additional points would be tertiary.

Once the treatment points have been located, the therapist proceeds through the remaining steps in the protocol, which are the same as those for the single-point protocol described in Chapter 9.

The multi-point protocol is another way to energetically map out and treat various psychological conditions. There are a number of alternative models that can be delineated, although I shall leave those explorations for another time. Presently we turn to another level of attunement and chunking, involving the energetic structure of core beliefs that can enhance or impair one's health and functioning.

Chapter 10

TRANSFORMING CORE BELIEFS

Belief like any other moving body follows the path of least resistance.

— *Samuel Butler*

MANY DSM-IV Axis I disorders, such as phobias, PTSD, anxiety, adjustment disorders, depression, respond quite well to single-point and multi-point protocols. However, when there exists an attendant Axis II personality disorder (e.g., dependent, paranoid, borderline, narcissistic) or a significantly limiting core belief (*I am essentially weak and incapable; others are out to get me; others will inevitably abandon me*), eventual relapse is generally the rule even when immediate relief is reported in the session. In such instances the core belief structure is so deeply ingrained and pervasive in its psychological-energetic topography that it ultimately degrades the therapeutic results.

While some instances of immediate and recurrent regression may be attributable to psychological reversal, too often this hypothesis leaves the therapist and client with little recourse save to chronically repeat psychological reversal and criteria-related reversal treatments in conjunction with the defined energy meridian treatment points, which may need to be repeatedly diagnosed. Here the therapist and client may go on a frustrating recursive hunt that ultimately demoralizes the client and undermines the "therapeutic" process due to limited gains.

Alternatively, it has been proposed that chronic relapse is predominantly the result of sensitivity to various exogenous substances, sometimes referred to as *energy toxins* (Callahan & Callahan, 1996). Essentially, the toxin is said to cause a resurgence of the symptoms and frequently psychological reversal as well. While in many instances this appears to be correct, frequently this position has played out clinically as a garbage pail concept that serves to shore up the model rather than assist the client toward achieving therapeutic results. Many clients, told that recalcitrance of their psychological problem is the result of energy toxic reactions to caffeine, corn, herbs, mushrooms, peas, rice, wheat, tomatoes, and so on, have been placed on ascetic diets to little or no benefit. No doubt in some instances such a restrictive diet will result in positive psychological changes as a result of any number of factors, including the fact that the diet is possibly healthier, as well as placebo effect and a sense of self-efficacy concomitant to having accomplished such an astronomical feat. In most instances, however, this hardly qualifies as an elegant solution to the client's presenting problem. On the other hand, being on a highly prohibitive diet can prove demoralizing to some clients, especially when the prohibitions result in little or no clinical improvement.

CORE BELIEFS PROTOCOL RATIONALE

Pragmatically the core beliefs protocol should be employed when the single-point and multi-point protocols do not achieve adequate results or when it is clinically obvious that the client's clinical condition and/or belief structure will interfere with achieving appreciable results. The guiding assumption of this protocol is that the energy disruptions at the basis of a psychological problem can be substantially treated by addressing the energy structure of the core belief or beliefs that underlie the psychological disorder. The protocol employs manual muscle testing to delineate the core belief and to therapy localize the active treatment point or points consistent with the energy structure of the belief. The client is then directed to physically stimulate the energy system at the localized site(s), thus removing the negative affects or emotions that drive the core belief and the psychological symptoms. It is assumed that there is a significant interface between the energy structure of the presenting symptom (e.g., depression) and the energy structure of the underlying belief-affect (e.g., belief that one is worthlessness). Assuming that the Axis I disorder is fundamentally subsumed by the Axis II disorder or belief structure, alleviation of the latter will frequently resolve the former as well. However, my clinical experience reveals that frequently the two aspects are sufficiently distinct, such that after the limiting core belief is addressed, the presenting symptom must be separately treated.

CORE BELIEFS PROTOCOL

Preparation

In addition to the usual preparation, as described in Chapter 2, I inform the client that it is often necessary to determine if there are underlying beliefs contributing to the psychological problem. Specifically, I educate the client about the guiding influence of negative core beliefs, or what might be called *mind-sets*, in terms of contributing to his or her experience of depression or anxiety. For example, I point out that if a person holds a long-term belief that he or she is essentially worthless, feelings of depression will understandably follow. A belief that one will inevitably be abandoned by significant others can also lead to depression, anxiety, and behaviors that can push others away and land one in acute care facilities. Additionally, I emphasize that the more energetically ingrained the belief, the more the person will tend to experience the belief as a fact rather than just a belief. This discussion begins the process of disentangling the client from the limiting core belief. The individual comes to stand back from the belief, to observe it rather than continue to be associated with it. This serves to weaken the energetic bond of the belief so that it becomes less attracting.

Introductory Statement

The core beliefs protocol might be introduced with the following low-key statement, which may be modified to suit the therapist's personal style. (Part of this statement has been given earlier [pp. 40–41].)

There are a lot of ideas about what causes emotional problems. Different people say it's stress, or stressful situations in your life, negative thoughts, or even chemical imbalance. I'm sure they are all right, because all these things work together. What's more, it seems that there is also an electrical part, kind of the switch that turns on the emotional problem. So if there is an awful situation in your life or something terrible happened, you might have certain thoughts or beliefs about it, and these in turn trigger electrical impulses in your brain and body that create an imbalance in your chemistry and produce the upsetting emotions like anxiety, depression, anger, and so on. And this all feeds back into the whole system and keeps it going.

Now, as far as the connection between beliefs and that electrical part are concerned, it seems that it can be tracked down by using a simple muscle checking procedure. You see, the muscles and nerves work together, so when you have an upsetting emotion, it causes a change in your muscles, too. Negative beliefs that we have about ourselves and our circumstances do that as well. The muscles tend to become firmer with positive thoughts, beliefs, and emotions, and somewhat loose with negative thoughts, beliefs, and emotions. It isn't that the muscles are really weak at such times, just that the electricity through the nerves gets interrupted so that the muscle momentarily relaxes some.

The method involves checking the firmness in a shoulder muscle while you hold your arm out straight (or the muscles in your fingers as you make a circle with your index finger and thumb, etc.). Then I have you verbalize various beliefs in order to determine which ones are relevant in your case. After we determine which beliefs apply, I have you touch certain places on your body, sort of circuit breakers, that tell us what to do next. This lets us know about places on your body where you need to tap with your fingers to shut off upsetting feelings associated with negative beliefs. This makes it possible to efficiently rid yourself of those limiting beliefs. I'll probably also ask you to do some other things, like saying certain phrases, moving your eyes in different directions, humming, counting, and other things. We really need to work together cooperatively in this if it's going to work. Would this all be okay with you?

Discussion

A sensible way to begin the process of tracking down the most relevant limiting core beliefs is by really listening to what the client has to say. That is, if the therapist listens with a clear mind — paying attention with true openness — the core beliefs will often become readily and obviously apparent. To accomplish this end, the therapist should not be distracted by assumptions about what the belief might be, how much one might find the belief distasteful, what diagnostic category might be assigned to the client, and so on. At such times it seems that the client simply tells us what we need to know, offering the vital information on a silver platter, so to speak. For example:

"I don't know. I just feel like something is missing in my life. Like *I'm not complete.*"
"Things aren't going right. *I'm really unhappy.*"
"It's hard for me to trust anyone. But basically that's because *people can't be trusted.*"

"There's lots of things I'd like to do, but *I just can't get motivated.*"

"I know that I should be able to ignore what my wife has to say at such times, but when she gets really angry, I'm afraid that she's going to leave me. And then I feel so deserted (i.e., My wife will *abandon me*)."

After getting a fairly clear sense of what the core beliefs might be, the therapist can employ manual muscle testing to corroborate these hypotheses. Similar to the other protocols involving manual muscle testing, a number of considerations must be taken into account to increase the chances of validity. Follow the steps of qualifying the indicator muscle, doing preliminary calibration tests, diagnosing and correcting neurologic disorganization and massive psychological reversal, and accessing the problem state as in the single-point protocol (pp. 165–167). Then move on to identifying core beliefs.

Core Beliefs Identification

At this point the therapist, in collaboration with the client, has a sense of what negative core beliefs might be operating in the client's life in specific contexts or across contexts. Additionally, it has been established that the client can be manually muscle tested and that MPR is not present. It is now time to manually muscle test for specific core beliefs.

Often it is useful to show the client a list of positive and negative core beliefs and to discuss which of these the client feels might be important in his or her life. In this regard Table 10.1, Selected Core Beliefs, can prove of value in identifying the beliefs.[1]

As a potential belief is identified, it can be subjected to manual muscle testing. This involves simply challenging the indicator muscle after the client states the positive counterpart of the negative core belief. For example, if the client seems to hold the belief of being unworthy, this can be tested further by having the client say, "I am worthy," after which the muscle is be tested. If the muscle tests weak, this suggests that the client does not hold this belief, and perhaps holds the opposite negative belief.

Next the indicator muscle is tested in response to the statement, "I am

---

[1] The examiner should note that Table 10.1 is not an exhaustive list. Depending on the individual client being evaluated, other relevant beliefs will be discoverable.

unworthy." If the muscle now tests strong, this further corroborates that this is a negative core belief held by the client.

The examiner should keep in mind that the client may hold a number of negative core beliefs that need to be identified before substantial personality change and/or change within the specific context for which therapy is being sought can be realized. Moreover, context-specific beliefs (e.g., I'll never get a good job; I won't make an adequate income) differ from global core beliefs (e.g., I'm inadequate; I'm a bad person) and that difference needs to be taken into account when conducting this diagnostic and therapeutic process.

Table 10.1
Selected Core Beliefs

POSITIVE BELIEFS	NEGATIVE BELIEFS
I am achieving.	I am not achieving.
I am appealing.	I am unappealing.
I am attractive.	I am unattractive.
I am capable.	I am incapable.
I am cherished.	I am/will be abandoned.
I am competent.	I am incompetent.
I am creative.	I am not creative.
I am deserving.	I am undeserving.
I am fortunate.	I am unfortunate.
I can get what I want.	I cannot get what I want.
I am good.	I am bad, evil.
I am healthy.	I am unhealthy, sick, ill.
I am honorable.	I am shameful.
I am innocent.	I am guilty.
I am intelligent.	I am unintelligent, stupid.
I am interesting.	I am uninteresting, dull.
I am likable.	I am not likable.
I am lovable.	I am unlovable.
I am loving.	I am not loving.
I am mentally healthy.	I am mentally ill, crazy.
I am motivated.	I am unmotivated.

(continued)

(Table 10.1 Continued)

I am not inferior.	I am inferior.
I am powerful.	I am powerless.
I am productive.	I am unproductive.
I am respectable.	I am not respectable.
I am respected.	I am not respected.
I am safe.	I am unsafe.
I am secure.	I am insecure.
I am smart.	I am stupid, dumb.
I am strong.	I am weak.
I am successful.	I am unsuccessful.
I can trust.	I cannot trust.
I am understanding.	I am not understanding.
I am understood.	I am misunderstood.
I am valuable.	I am valueless, worthless.
I am warm.	I am cold.
I am worthy.	I am unworthy, inadequate.
I am worthwhile.	I am not worthwhile.

Scaling

The desired positive core belief can be scaled for the sake of obtaining ongoing clinical feedback while the core beliefs protocol is being conducted. One approach is to define a continuum from the negative to the positive (e.g., unlovable → lovable), with 0 at the negative end of the continuum (e.g., unlovable) and 10 at the positive end (e.g., totally lovable). The client indicates a positive belief score (PBS) from 0–10, and the indicator muscle is tested to corroborate the stated rating. Intermittently throughout the treatment, the PBS is obtained in order to guide the process.

Psychological Reversal

Psychological and criteria-related reversals can block the client's disengagement from a negative core belief. Once the specific negative core belief has been identified and the client basically understands the concept of reversal, the therapist can test for reversal and make the necessary corrections. For example, if the client globally believes that he or she is a bad person, manual muscle testing can be conducted with test statements for various reversals, including the following:

Specific: "I want to believe that I'm not a bad person (or I'm a good person)" vs. "I want to continue to believe that I'm a bad person."

Deep level: "I will believe that I'm not a bad person" vs. "I will continue to believe that I'm a bad person."

Possibility: "It's possible for me to believe that I'm not a bad person" vs. "It is not possible for me to believe that I'm not a bad person."

Identity: "If I no longer believe that I'm a bad person, I'll lose an important part of my identity" vs. "If I no longer believe that I'm a bad person, I will not lose an important part of my identity."

In order to temporarily remove the reversal so that treatments specifically directed at the belief can work, the following respective treatment statements can be used in conjunction with acupoint stimulation:

Specific: "I deeply accept myself even though I believe that I'm a bad person."

Deep level: "I deeply accept myself even if I never believe that I'm a good person."

Possibility: "I deeply accept myself even if it isn't possible for me to believe that I'm a good person."

Identity: "I deeply accept myself even if I lose an important part of my identity by believing that I'm not a bad person."

Often the issue will be deeper than simply wanting to believe that one is not a bad person, worthless, inadequate, or whatever the essence of the negative core belief might be. If the client has convincing enough "evidence" that he or she is bad or incompetent, for example, the correction may not be as straightforward as coming to hold a belief in stark opposition to the history that supports it. Such a position might be experienced by some as akin to delusion or negative hallucination. Here we are obviously in the realm of *identity*. The correction should initially focus on the issue of the client wanting to *be* or *become* competent or wanting to *be* or *to become* a good person. The examiner might use test statements such as the following:

Specific:	"I want to be (or become) a good person (competent, etc.)" vs. "I don't want to be (or become) a good person (competent, etc.)"
Deep level:	"I will become a good person (competent, etc.)" vs. "I will not become a good person (competent, etc.)"
Possibility:	"It's possible for me to become a good person (competent, etc.)" vs. "It is impossible for me to become a good person (competent, etc.)"
Identity:	"I'll lose an important part of my identity if I become a good person (competent, etc.)" vs. "I will not lose an important part of my identity if I become a good person (competent, etc.)"

Respective corrections would be as follows:

Specific:	"I deeply accept myself even though I'm a bad person (incompetent, etc.)"
Deep level:	"I deeply accept myself even if I never become a good person (competent, etc.)"
Possibility:	"I deeply accept myself even if it isn't possible for me to become a good person (competent, etc.)"
Identity:	"I deeply accept myself even if I lose an important part of my identity if I become a good person (competent, etc.)"

Resonance Locking the Negative Core Belief

After the negative core belief has been attuned, often it will continue to resonate for a sufficient period of time so that the remainder of the diagnostic protocol can be completed. However, we cannot be assured of this, since intervening thoughts and environmental stimuli may degrade the signal strength and interfere with accurate diagnosis. This may be a function of the degree to which the client is able consciously to access the belief field, or perhaps it speaks of the client's skill at repression. Continuation of resonance can be insured by employing resonance locking procedures such as the leg lock or the glabella tap, as described on pages 115–118.

Therapy Localization and Stimulation

After the client has attuned the belief and a resonance lock has been established, the therapist guides the client through the hemisphere dominance test, as described on pages 103–104. Then the therapist continues with the remaining steps of the single-point protocol, therapy localizing alarm and treatment points, and stimulating those points.

Even though the belief is in resonance lock, it may be helpful to have the client regularly verbalize or think about the positive core belief during the process, preferably with the intention of accepting the belief (e.g., "I am worthwhile"). The therapist may also find it necessary to stimulate several points, similar to the multi-point protocol. After several points have been found, the client taps or touches the points one after another for several seconds while holding the desired belief in mind.

Ongoing Evaluation

Intermittently a PBS should be taken, sometimes corroborated by manual muscle testing. As long as the PBS has increased by at least two points with each evaluation, stimulation of the treatment point is resumed until the PBS is within the range of 8–10.

If the PBS stops increasing, the therapist should check for and correct any intervening reversal before continuing stimulation. Possible reversals at this point include the specific version (i.e., "I want to *completely* believe . . ."), deep level (i.e., "I will *completely* believe . . ."), or any alternative criteria-related reversal (i.e., those addressing deserving, safety, possibility, motivation, deprivation, etc.). If a specific intervening reversal is not revealed, the therapist may choose to check for the most common criteria that may intervene to block treatment progress, trust his/her intuition, or evaluate with a screening statement such as, "There is another reversal blocking the resolution of this problem."

Evaluating Results

When the PBS is at 10, or has otherwise stopped increasing and a reversal is not involved, it is time for one of the balancing procedures: nine gamut treatments, brain balancing procedure, or cross-crawl exercises.

Reevaluation and Further Treatment

Then the therapist once again checks the PBS and corroborates via muscle testing. If the PBS is not within the 8–10 range, and a reversal is not present, the therapist again diagnoses any other meridian imbalance. That is, the

HDT → alarm point localization → treatment point localization protocol is repeated.

When the PBS is within 8–10 range, the therapist introduces either the floor-to-ceiling eye roll (ER) or the elaborated eye roll (EER) in order to alleviate any remaining stress and solidify results.

The indicator muscle generally weakens when a non-incorporated positive belief is attuned. In such instances, therapy localization of an active treatment point results in a strengthening of the indicator muscle while the subject attunes the positive belief. After the positive belief has been incorporated, the indicator muscle should remain strong when the subject verbalizes ownership of the belief, with or without therapy localization of the treatment point. If therapy localizing the treatment point now results in weakening of the indicator muscle, the treatment point is still active and there is still stress in the system, indicating that the positive belief has not been wholly incorporated. Therefore, additional treatment directed at that point is needed. Once the belief is incorporated, the indicator muscle will remain strong with and without therapy localization of the point, and repeating the HDT will reveal a strong indicator muscle while evaluating either hemisphere.

Validation and Assignments

It is unusual for a single treatment of this nature to result in lasting elimination and transformation of the negative belief. When a thought-energy structure has achieved the status of a negative core belief, its tentacles extend into many aspects and contexts of the person's life. Therefore many layers of the proverbial onion will need to be peeled away. Several therapeutic sessions and client-administered in vivo repetitions of the treatments will often be needed to dismiss the negative belief and solidly establish the positive one. The patient should be debriefed accordingly and taught how to repeat the treatments between sessions to insure incorporation of the healthier core belief structure.

A SIMPLIFIED CORE BELIEF PROTOCOL

The core belief protocol is a sophisticated and comprehensive way to address core and other beliefs. Prior to approaching beliefs in this fashion, the therapist may find it convenient to attempt a more simplistic approach. After the negative belief (e.g., "I'm not worthy; I can't learn algebra") has been diagnosed via discussion and manual muscle testing, a positive alternative belief is specified (e.g., "I am worthwhile; I enjoy learning algebra with ease"). Any psychological reversals are then corrected and the negative affect erasing method (NAEM) is used to discharge the negative belief. After manual muscle testing demonstrates that the negative belief is not operating, the positive belief is instilled with NAEM. Specifically, the client rehearses the positive belief in his/her mind while stimulating the NAEM treatment points. Often the instillation process can be done by simply stimulating the third eye point (GV-24.5) or the gamut spot (TE-3). The client is told to repeat the procedure regularly until the positive belief has been integrated.

Chapter 11

BLOCKS TO TREATMENT EFFECTIVENESS III: ENERGY TOXINS

Shame can occur when our secrets are exposed, when an
aberration of biology produces an atypical depression,
or when we ingest certain chemicals.

— *Donald L. Nathanson*, Shame and Pride

MANY PATIENTS CAN BE ASSISTED in alleviating various psychological problems by employing NAEM, HELP, single-point or multi-point protocols, with some requiring primary or attendant treatment of various dysfunctional core beliefs. Yet others will evidence a recalcitrant tendency for the primary symptoms to be resurrected or to resist treatment efforts altogether. In many such instances, an exogenous substance may be the culprit. That is, various substances may significantly disrupt the bioenergy system, either preventing other treatments from working or otherwise resulting in a degradation of positive results upon exposure to the exogenous substance. Practically, any substance is capable of having a toxic effect, not merely the more obvious ones such as alcohol, caffeine, cat dander, corn, decongestants, herbs, laundry detergent, mold, nicotine, perfume, pollen, wheat, and so forth. Also, the effects of energy toxins are often quite idiosyncratic, consistent with the old adage, "One man's meat is another man's poison."

193

ALLERGIES AND HYPERSENSITIVITY

If one suspects *allergy* or *hypersensitivity*, it is essential to determine which substances are blocking treatment effectiveness and to either prevent exposure to the substances or, when possible, neutralize the effects of those substances. The assessment phase of this process generally begins by treating the patient and then having him/her record when the psychological disturbance returns. An *exposure diary* is useful in this regard. Such a diary includes detailed information concerning dates and times of meals, snacks, various activities such as lawn mowing, exposure to perfumes, excessive temperatures, psychosocial stress, etc., as well as the precise times when psychological symptoms were noticed. This gives the therapist and patient detailed information as a basis for further investigation through manual muscle tests and for management and treatment procedures.

Before detailing the diagnostic and treatment methods specific to this area, it should be noted that while some use allergen and *energy toxin* synonymously, in the strictest sense these terms are not equivalent. An allergy may be defined as

> an altered reaction of body tissues to a specific substance which . . . in nonsensitive persons will, in similar amounts, produce no effect. It is essentially an antibody-antigen reaction but in some cases the antibody cannot be demonstrated. The reaction may be due to the release of histamine, or histamine-like substances from injured cells. (Thomas, 1973, p. A-55)

An allergy is therefore a certain kind of immune system response to an allergen. In essence, the response is a misinterpretation within the immune system's communication network. That is, the immune system mistakenly identifies the substance as if it is a dangerous invader, such as a bacterium or a virus. Once the individual is sensitized to the antigen, in most instances the dysfunctional immune response becomes chronic:

> When exposed to allergens, allergic individuals develop an excess of an antibody called immunoglobulin E (IgE). The IgE antibodies react with allergens to release histamines and other chemicals from cell tissues that produce various allergic symptoms. In other words, the immune system mistakenly identifies harmless substances as dangerous invaders and activates antibodies to defend the body. The development

of an allergy begins with sensitization to the substance on first contact, usually without symptoms. A second exposure to the substance, however, allows the previously created antibodies to become active and produce symptoms. (Cutler, 1997, p. 3)[1]

Hypersensitivity, on the other hand, refers to noxious effects of a substance; it is not classified as an allergic reaction. When the substance is observed to disrupt one's bioenergy system, it is also referred to as an energy toxin. In some instances the exogenous substance may also cause a recognizable allergic reaction (e.g., runny nose, itchy eyes, hives), although this is not invariably the case. In many cases an allergic reaction or hypersensitivity results in an energy imbalance as well, but an energy toxin does not necessarily result in a perceivable allergic reaction or other more common symptoms of hypersensitivity.

When a substance results in an energy toxic effect, the energy system evidences an imbalance such that generally effective therapeutic methods are blocked or impaired in their ability to alleviate the psychological problem. The energy toxin causes a recurrent reversal and neurologic disorganization, blocking other efforts to balance the energy system and remove the subtle energy codes within the thought field (i.e., perturbations). One way to circumvent this effect is to avoid exposure to the substance for a sufficient period of time, from a few days to as much as a couple months, so that treatments specifically directed at the presenting psychological symptoms can be effective. After the psychological problem has been eliminated, the person may eventually be able to consume or be exposed to the substance without experiencing a relapse of symptoms. However, this is often ill-advised, since exposure to the toxin may result in other untoward effects, including negatively affecting one's health and blocking therapeutic effectiveness in other areas for which the patient may seek treatment.

In addition, some substances have been observed to independently trigger negative emotional symptoms. For example, pseudoephedrine, a compound used in many cold remedies, can mimic the effects of adrenaline and promote a sense of anxiety. Many people are also familiar with the so-called caffeine jitters. Other medications, especially certain antihypertensive preparations, can elicit chronic feelings of guilt or shame.

---

[1]Rochlitz (1995), a physicist who has developed energetic means for the treatment of allergies, points out that other classes of immunoglobulins, including IgA, IgD, IgG, and IgM, can produce antibody-antigen complexes.

People who take medication to reduce high blood pressure, especially those drugs that decrease our sensitivity to the neurotransmitter *norepinephrine*, are likely to complain of "depression." Questioned closely, these patients seem to have a disorder of guilt, telling us that they have done something bad for which they should be punished even when they "know" they have not. Early in the era of experimentation that led to the development of the antihypertensive drugs, patients were given a chemical compound called *alphamethylparatyrosine* — a compound that resembles the amino acid *tyrosine*, one normally found in the body and which is important in the manufacture of norepinephrine. Although the patients given this compound were described only as "depressed," monkeys given the same medication were seen as socially withdrawn, unable to make facial contact with each other, likely to sit with bowed head and averted gaze. It is commonly said that these chemicals are interfering with the circuitry for normal mood, but I think they do this by producing an internal experience that can only be interpreted by the organism in terms of the innate affect shame. (Nathanson, 1992, pp. 146–147)

It should be noted that energy toxins are not limited to inhalant and ingested substances or dermatological irritants. A number of other environmental factors can be energy toxic, causing recurrent reversals and neurologic disorganization, interfering with treatment effects. Assuming that the body possesses a subtle bioenergy system that has electromagnetic characteristics, it is probable that other energy sources, such as high tension wires, microwave ovens, and computer monitors, can exert a similar negative effect (Becker, 1990). Similarly, Diamond (1980b, 1985) has discussed the negative effects on life energy of florescent lights, quartz watches, and even certain kinds of music.

Considering all of the energy toxic effects simultaneously occurring all around and through us, we can assume that they play a significant role in a whole range of modern-day illnesses, including a number of mental health disorders. Many have recognized that chemical substances can elicit negative reactions, including attention deficit disorders, that may be incorrectly assumed to be fundamentally psychologically or neurologically based (Nathanson, 1992; Rapp, 1986, 1991; Walther, 1988). Of great concern is the fact that while we are exposed to thousands of new substances every year, most have not been tested for their effects on behavior (Travis, McLean, & Ribar, 1989).

TESTING PROCEDURES

Assuming that certain substances can interfere with therapy and even cause negative emotional and behavioral reactions, how can we diagnose their presence and institute measures to minimize their effects? As previously mentioned, one of the essential tools of the energy therapist is the exposure diary, in which the patient maintains an ongoing record of foods and beverages consumed, various activities, etc., in addition to times of symptoms, such as mood changes or cognitive disorganization. This provides a means of temporally correlating emotional responses with foods and other substance exposures.

Table 11.1 shows a portion of an exposure diary. In this example, we have to ask what is causing the individual's anxiety. The person might generally assume that it had something to do with his drive to work, the stress of arriving at work, being aware of the agenda for the day, the content of the letter dictated or the conversation with Jack. While these are all reasonable possibilities, it is also plausible that the reaction was triggered by something eaten at breakfast such as the coffee, sugar, orange juice, or corn flakes. It is also possible that the nervousness was secondary to the aftershave or the soap or shampoo used during the shower. Any other substances that the person consumed, inhaled, or was exposed to in other ways could have caused the reaction. But which one(s)?

Table 11.1
Exposure Diary

TIME	ACTIVITY	EMOTIONAL REACTION
7–7:15 AM	Shower	
7:15–7:30	Shave and dress	
7:30–7:45	Coffee, corn flakes, milk, sugar, orange juice	
7:45–8:00	Drive to work	
8:00	Arrive at work, coffee Review agenda	Nervous (level 5)
8:30–8:45	Dictating letter	Nervous (level 7)
9:00–9:30	Talk with Jack	Nervous (level 8)

In order to answer this question, the therapist and patient might first compile a list of the various exposures: the coffee at home, refined sugar, orange juice, milk, corn flakes, aftershave, bar soap, shampoo, hair spray, the coffee at work (might be a different brand), etc. At this point each of the substances can be assessed via the protocol below:

ENERGY TOXIN DIAGNOSTIC PROTOCOL (ETDP)

1. Qualify a strong indicator muscle.
2. Calibrate and test in the clear.
3. Subject pronounces the name of the substance (for example, "Brand X perfume"), after which the indicator muscle is again challenged.
4. If the muscle weakens at this point, the substance is likely an energy toxin. This may be further corroborated by having the subject smell the substance or hold the substance at each of the following locations while testing the indicator muscle: navel, temples, hips, and upper sternum. Weakening of the indicator muscle suggests that the substance is energy toxic to the subject.
5. If the muscle does not weaken after the subject says the name of the substance or run the additional tests cited, it *may not* be an energy toxin. Evaluate further as indicated below.
6. Initially have subject say, "I want to be healthy," followed by, "I want to be ill." This is followed by challenging the muscle, thus checking for a *massive health reversal*. If a health reversal is present, at least temporarily correct for this in any way that works (e.g., subject massages neurolymphatic reflex on left side of chest while stating, "I deeply and profoundly accept myself even though I have this problem").
7. Assuming that a massive health reversal is not present, next have the subject say, "(*Name of substance*), I want to be healthy" (e.g., "*Corn*, I want to be healthy.") After the subject makes this statement, the muscle is again tested. This procedure not only tests for when the substance is an energy toxin, but also determines if the person has adversely accommodated to the substance, a profound reversal (e.g., reversal of the body morality). If the muscle tests strong, assuming a valid test, the substance is not an energy toxin. As an additional check, the muscle can again be challenged after the subject says, "(*Name of substance*), I want to be sick." In the latter instance, the muscle should test weak.

8.   Assuming a valid test, if the indicator muscle weakens after the subject
     says, "(*Name of substance*), I want to be healthy," the substance is an
     energy toxin. The opposite statement can be tested for corroboration
     (i.e., "(*Name of substance*), I want to be sick").

The energy toxin diagnostic protocol (ETDP) is distinct from other muscle
testing procedures for assessing energy toxins in that it also takes into account
the possibility of a massive health reversal. The relevance of this factor is
twofold. First, the presence of such a reversal is significant in and of itself.
If the patient is intrinsically oriented toward illness, this surely deserves close
attention. We might want to know what events and factors led to this state
of affairs. Was it a trauma from which the patient has not recovered? If it
was a trauma, was a dysfunctional core belief (e.g., "My health is shot")
installed at that time? Is it the result of a negative dictum from a significant
person in the person's life (e.g., "You're the most unhealthy person I know"
or "The good die young")? Protocols presented earlier in this text should
prove helpful in this area.

Second, if we do not evaluate for the presence of the massive health
reversal, it may be concealed within the test phrase, "(*Name of substance*),
I want to be healthy." That is, one could unconsciously solely focus in on
the "*I want to be healthy*," overlooking the name of the substance in each
instance, while the roster of energy toxins accumulates. In such instances,
the therapist might erroneously advise the patient to go on a highly restrictive,
depriving diet, instructing the patient to avoid practically everything under
the sun.

BUT WHICH TOXIN?

Once the substances that are energy toxic to the patient have been identified,
how do we know which one or ones are responsible for blocking the effectiveness of treatment? It should be borne in mind that, while a patient may
demonstrate toxicity to a number of substances, not all of them will necessarily be responsible for impeding progress or causing regression in the area
targeted for therapeutic intervention. Some toxins may not disrupt the bioenergy as significantly as others. Some may specifically interfere with treatment
for depression, while others may block successful treatment with respect to
anxiety, anger, feelings of guilt, etc. This is possibly a function of a meridian-
toxin interface. In the same way that certain muscles and emotions appear
to be associated with specific meridians, substances may be similarly associ-

ated. This is another factor that needs to be taken into account so as to not place the patient on an unnecessarily restrictive diet. A little additional refinement in the diagnostic protocol makes it possible to more closely pinpoint the most relevant impediments.

COPING WITH HYPERSENSITIVITY AND ALLERGIES

An obvious way to deal with substances that cause allergic reactions, hypersensitivity, and energy disruptions is to avoid them altogether. In some cases this is the only recourse, especially when the substance tends invariably to result in significant reactions and methods designed to neutralize the effects of the substance prove ineffective. It should be noted that at times the negative substance reaction is really in the person's best interest.

> For example, one may have an intolerance to milk that is considered an allergy; instead it is a genetic lack of lactase, causing inability to break down lactose. When treating allergies, one should consider if the reaction has a beneficial purpose for the individual. (Walther, 1988, p. 499)

In many instances the aversive effects of substances are a function of threshold, the accumulation of the substance in one's body being the significant variable. In this instance one option is to avoid the substance until one has been adequately detoxified, usually within a few weeks. After this time, the patient may be able to tolerate occasional exposure to the substance without incurring untoward effects. In the case of foods, the patient may be advised to follow a rotary diet, such that the food is consumed no more than once every four days (Rapp, 1991). A dietary regime of this nature helps to further clarify if the patient can tolerate the food. When the patient is able to consume the food at this frequency, he/she can also prevent toxic reactions by lowering the level of accumulation on an ongoing basis. This kind of regime is especially relevant for patients who experience allergic or other toxic effects to a large number of foods.

DETOXIFICATION

If the patient appears to have an accumulation of toxins in his or her system, which can have profound health and mental health implications, detoxification may be needed. Rapp (1991) advises patients to drink plenty of purified water and also offers a number of other suggestions for accelerating detoxification, such as the consumption of antioxidants. A number of nutritionists and therapists have praised the benefits of an organic sulfur compound, methylsulfonylmethane (MSM), also an antioxidant, with regard to its capacity to promote detoxification and other health benefits. Its chemical formula is $(CH^3)2SO^2$. MSM apparently makes cell walls more permeable, facilitating nutrition and the alleviation of toxins from cells. For years it has been used as a dietary supplement for animals and more recently for humans. It is reported to promote healing and to be of benefit for a wide range of conditions, including allergies, arthritis, and asthma. This organic sulfur, not to be confused with sulfa drugs, is the fourth most prevalent mineral in the human body and is found in all vegetable and animal life. The MSM on the market is primarily vegetable derived.

ENERGY TOXIN NEUTRALIZATION PROTOCOLS

Even though energy toxins can interfere with treatment effectiveness, there are frequently times when the toxic level is sufficiently reduced, allowing for the treatment to work. Consequently, it is not always necessary to manage toxins intentionally if the patient is diligent in the practice of assigned treatments. Admittedly this is a big IF, and if toxins do result in profound psychological reversal, the reversed patient, by definition, would not be inclined to practice the treatments. That is, why do something that is good for you when your unconscious commitment is in the opposite direction?[2] Therefore, having a method available to desensitize the patient to the energy toxin is important in many cases.

Several methods have been reported to permanently desensitize patients to allergens and energy toxins. Hallbom and Smith (1988) demonstrate a method based in neuro-linguistic programming that involves dissociation and other components. This method appears to be based on the position that the immune system evidences a stress reaction when the allergen is present. By having the patient imagine consuming the substance while engaged in therapeutic dissociation, the stress reaction is alleviated and the

[2]This is especially a problem with substance-dependent patients, since the substances to which they are addicted are frequently energy toxic as well, if only because of the level of accumulation in the system. In cases of drug and alcohol dependence, abstinence is judiciously preferred to attempting desensitization of the patient to the energy toxic effects of the substance.

circuit breakers, so to speak, are reset. The method is similar to the NLP method for treating phobias and traumas, visual/kinesthetic dissociation.

Nambudripad (1993) has developed a method based on acupuncture and applied kinesiology, the Nambudripad Allergy Elimination Technique (NAET), for which she reports high success. Cutler (1997) reports on the effectiveness of Nambudripad's method in conjunction with enzyme therapy. Fleming (1996) initially worked with NAET and later developed her own method, for which she also reports high success in treating allergies as well as psychological trauma.

I have also developed a couple of protocols that have been effective in neutralizing energy toxins and allergens. While these protocols can be applied by the therapist, it is also useful to educate the patient in the treatment aspects of the protocols, since practice between therapy sessions is usually needed. These protocols are not recommended for the treatment of allergens from which the patient has experienced severe allergic reactions, such as anaphylactic shock. Any attempts to utilize these protocols in such cases should only be conducted by health care professionals with expertise in this area. These protocols are offered primarily for the treatment of energy toxins that impair psychotherapeutic success.

Energy Toxin Neutralization Protocol No. 1

1. Conduct ETDP to determine what substances are toxic to the patient.
2. Diagnose and correct any reversals that may be present.
3. Patient thinks about the identified toxin while doing a global energy balancing method such as the negative affect erasing method (NAEM) or over-energy correction for approximately one minute.
4. Test indicator muscle again while patient thinks about the substance. If there is a strong muscle response, this suggests that a correction has occurred. If the response is weak, this suggests that the correction has not occurred. In this instance, repeating the global balancing for a longer period of time may prove effective; otherwise go to the second protocol.
5. If the muscle response was strong, test the substance again by having the patient smell the substance or hold the substance at each of the following locations while the indicator muscle is tested: navel, temples, hips, and upper sternum. Weakening of the indicator muscle suggests that the substance is still energy toxic to the patient. A strong indicator muscle response suggests that the substance has been desensitized.
6. If the substance tests as desensitized, the patient is instructed to avoid

the substance for 25 hours and drink at lease eight glasses of pure water during that time period.
7. Reevaluate after that time period has elapsed.

Energy Toxin Neutralization Protocol No. 2

1. Conduct ETDP to determine what substances are toxic to the patient.
2. Diagnose and correct any reversals that may be present.
3. Patient thinks about or verbalizes the identified toxin while index and middle fingers of left hand are positioned immediately under the navel.
4. With fingers and thumb of right hand the patient briskly rubs the neurolymphatic reflexes located on either side of the sternum and between the second and third ribs.
5. With the fingers of the left hand still positioned under the navel, the patient taps on the left gamut spot (TE-3) while doing the elaborated eye roll (EER).
6. After completing the EER, the patient stimulates both K-27 points by tapping or rubbing for several seconds.
7. Patient now switches hands and repeats steps 3 through 6.
8. Test indicator muscle again while patient thinks about the substance. If there is a strong muscle response, this suggests that a correction has occurred. If the response is weak, this suggests that the correction has not occurred. In this instance repeating the method again may prove effective; otherwise, consider another method of addressing the toxin.
9. If the muscle response was strong, test the substance again by having the patient smell the substance or hold the substance at the navel, temples, hips, and upper sternum while the indicator muscle is tested. Weakening of the indicator muscle suggests that the substance is still energy toxic to the patient. A strong indicator muscle response suggests that the substance has been desensitized.
10. If the substance tests as desensitized, the patient is instructed to avoid the substance for 25 hours and drink at least eight glasses of pure water during that time period.
11. Reevaluate after that time period has elapsed.

Usually energy toxins do not pose a problem in terms of diagnosis and treatment of psychological problems. However, it is important that the psychotherapist be aware of the possible interfering effects of toxins and of the various ways to address them. There are certainly occasions in which a toxin is the principal cause of the psychological condition, such as with certain allergic reactions and affect-stimulating medications. In such cases psychotherapy will not be effective unless the substance is identified and eliminated or neutralized, and frequently psychotherapy is not even necessary. Often these patients report a wide array of sensitivities, including sensitivity to psychotropic medications. A health care practitioner trained in allergy and environmental medicine is often a beneficial consultant in such cases.

Chapter 12

THE FUTURE OF
ENERGY PSYCHOLOGY

> It is possible to believe that all the past is but the beginning
> of a beginning, and that all that is and has been is but the twilight
> of the dawn. It is possible to believe that all the human mind has
> ever accomplished is but the dream before the awakening.
>
> —H. G. Wells

A BOOK IS NEVER COMPLETE, merely released. As it is being written, many attractive avenues become visible, and yet the project at hand needs to be completed before exploring those other paths; otherwise, the book would never be available. In this final chapter, I touch upon some issues that will affect the future of energy psychology.

PARADIGM SHIFT

This work represents a practical approach to the diagnosis and treatment of psychological problems and elaborates a distinct paradigm for the fields of psychology and psychotherapy. In many respects psychology is still in a pre-paradigmatic phase, judging by the multitude of theories and the field's impetus to model itself after the natural sciences (Giorgi, 1970). Psychology, both a natural science and a human one,[1] is still searching for a paradigm

---

[1] In a sense the natural sciences are also human sciences, if we accept the premise that there is no true separation of subject and object. The very fact that the natural sciences are created by people brings our consciousness into play, and thus even mathematics and physics become human sciences.

that suits its subject matter, human experience and behavior. What I offer here is only a humble beginning of an attempt to point the way toward an integration of natural and human science.

While suggesting that psychological problems can be conceptualized and treated energetically, we must bear in mind that this is merely a standpoint, a place to enter the system. Human experience has many dimensions. At a fundamental level, alteration of the energetic structure will often resolve the problem. However, thorough transformation is multidimensional and occurs at several interrelated levels. In no way does the specified psychological problem signify the whole of the individual's experience and functioning. Nevertheless, we might conceive of natural science dimensions in holographic terms; then, perhaps the structure of the energy field configuration is sufficiently fundamental to contain the whole of the dimensions that have been isolated, as well as others as yet to be defined. That is, the cognitive, neurologic, muscular, and chemical aspects of the disturbance can be subsumed energetically, although as functioning or dysfunction significantly congeals at more material or inertial levels, transformation initiated at the energy level necessarily entails a degree of inertial delay. And, unfortunately, there are some conditions that are so profoundly congealed that it is unlikely that contemporary energetic treatments will produce appreciable results. These anomalies are welcomed since they offer opportunities to further advance our models and understandings.

And there is still that wonderfully human dimension with which to "contend." The individual's experience and the meaning he or she gives to the problem and the resolution of the problem are dimensions that cannot be described in reductionistic terms. At this level something more than transmutation of electromagnetic configurations occurs. Moreover, this human dimension cannot be separated from the whole of the condition and its resolution. The interaction with a therapist in the process of identifying and alleviating the problem is also not easily compartmentalized, although protocols can be offered that assist the therapist-client toward interacting in ways that are beneficial.

Most psychotherapists interact with their clients around a number of themes. Certainly any effective therapist maintains rapport, instills motivation, explores expectations, offers useful reframes, negotiates, and employs a number of effective techniques and protocols to assist the patient in achieving outcomes. For example, the therapist learns to listen for specific limiting beliefs and then has various cognitive tools in his or her repertoire to expose the belief, challenge it, reframe it, and replace it. The guiding assumption is that psychological problems are a manifestation of such dysfunctional beliefs, and that if they can be altered, the patient will be further down the road toward cure. Thus the therapist is guided by a theoretical position and a methodology in which is nested a variety of techniques. As the theory and practice are explored in greater depth, refinements in methodology, protocols, and techniques emerge. These refinements develop since the initial procedures that emanated from the theory did not adequately produce the desired results. Also, different techniques develop for ulterior reasons, such as boredom on the part of the therapist or perhaps some ego considerations that have little to do with the advancement of the paradigm itself.

Theory does not always precede procedures. Sometimes techniques develop first and then the theory is built around them, which in turn generates other techniques and procedures. Nonetheless, in time it becomes clear that any model has limits. This is inevitable in view of the fact that models are merely representations of reality and not reality itself. They entail rules that attempt to organize different facts into some sort of a congruent and convenient whole. The process of developing models entails excluding certain data, developing generalizations about the data being utilized, and even distorting that data somewhat. The goal is to account for specific phenomena, to make predictions, and to achieve specific results. A model or paradigm will succeed to the extent that it effectively explains and makes predictions in ways that other models do not. However, there are always other factors involved, such as inertia and politics.

Max Planck was known for saying that a new paradigm is accepted only when the old guard has passed on. This speaks of the conservative nature of us all. Even the most liberal are conservative in their liberalism. We human beings are inclined to resist change once specific patterns or models have been incorporated into our ways of functioning. Surely this has something to do with our neurology as well as with energetic factors such as morphogenic fields and morphic resonance. In addition, there are ego issues involved. Once a commitment to a certain model has been made, a number of social and economic territorial issues come into play.

It seems that the way scientific and other models develop mimics the way individual minds come into being. While some may contend that there is only one Mind, in point of fact there are individual minds as well. A chip off the old block is still a chip and not the whole block. Once we come to develop a mind, we tend to keep it. More accurately, it often tends to keep us. Paradigmatic shifts become possible once the limits of the model have become increasingly too evident to ignore any longer and after we are able to step back from the model and see it for what it is: simply a model. People change their minds similarly.

As Thomas Kuhn (1962) pointed out nearly four decades ago, the scientific paradigm is maintained and advanced through the process of a dialectic between progressive and conservative powers. The assumptions of the established paradigm, which is really the opinion of the scientific aristocracy of the time, are vigorously defended, often by suppressing novelty, since the deviation is subversive. However, novelty cannot be suppressed for long. Anomalies demand our attention. And thus a scientific revolution is inevitable. As Hegel clarified long ago, the clash of thesis and antithesis results in the birth of a synthesis that possesses characteristics of both of its parents.

HISTORY REPEATING

Energy psychology developed within a particular context. In 1964, after studying *Muscles: Testing and Function* (Kendall & Kendall, 1949) and a wide array of other developments, George Goodheart, Jr., began the process of carving out a distinct discipline, applied kinesiology (see Gallo, 1998; Goodheart, 1987). Certification training in this professional field has been made available to chiropractic, osteopathic, and other physicians, psychologists, and others with licenses to diagnose. The governing body is the International College of Applied Kinesiology. Since applied kinesiology represents a significant departure from standard practice, it is really just beginning to have a significant impact on chiropractic and related disciplines. There is still considerable resistance to its acceptance.

Synthesizing a number of procedures from early applied kinesiology, John Thie (1973) developed *Touch for Health* for the health professional as well as the layperson. The goal of TFH has been to make energy balancing for health more widely available. In this way it has been the hope that individuals would employ these methods for preventative purposes, to help maintain energy balance. Although TFH is not professionally oriented in the way that the applied kinesiology literature is, it has perhaps had the greatest impact in tipping the scales in the direction of the applied kinesiology paradigm. At this point millions of copies of *Touch for Health*, Thie's seminal work, are in circulation.

In the meantime, Alan Beardall, a protégé of Goodheart, developed *clinical kinesiology*, evolving the practice of muscle testing to include an increasing number of muscles and adding other techniques such as the leg lock and use of hand modes or mudras to access information from the bio-computer. He also developed Nutri-West® Core-Level™ nutrients to balance out the chemical aspect of the *triad of health*. Like applied kinesiology, clinical kinesiology has catered to professionals, although aspects of the methodology have migrated throughout the kinesiology industry.

In time other kinesiological approaches sprung from these roots. *Three in One Concepts* or *One Brain* was developed by Gorden Stokes and Daniel Whiteside beginning in 1972. One Brain entails extensive muscle testing toward the goal of balancing the body and the mind at conscious and unconscious levels. Elaborate attunement is employed to pinpoint the origins and emotional features of the problem, asking the body via indicator muscle checking. Stress diffusion is a primary impetus in the treatment of psychological and learning problems (Holdway, 1995).

Also in 1972, John Barton developed *biokinesiology*. This method employs elaborate muscle testing to determine the emotional and nutritional needs of the person. Treatments include stress diffusion, nutrition, and biokinetic exercises (Holdway, 1995).

Psychologist Jimmy Scott's *health kinesiology* was developed in the late 1970s. This method is rooted in the Chinese five elements theory and over-energy in meridians. Treatment modalities include many procedures from applied kinesiology and Touch for Health, as well as herbs, homeopathic remedies, flower essences, gems, crystals, etc. (La Tourelle & Courtenay, 1992; Scott, 1988).

After studying TFH in 1979, Paul and Gail Dennison developed *educational kinesiology* or *Edu-K*, which emphasizes energetic and other TFH techniques for learning enhancement and amelioration of learning problems. Techniques include laterality repatterning, which involves cross-crawl and homolateral crawl in combination with eye movements and humming to enhance brain processing/coordination (Holdway, 1995).

Also after studying and being effectively treated with TFH, physicist Steven Rochlitz developed *human ecology balancing* in the early 1980s. This method employs a range of procedures from applied kinesiology and TFH, including manual muscle testing and methods specifically developed by Rochlitz, to treat allergies, asthma, arthritis, eczema, learning disorders, and a variety of other health problems (Rochlitz, 1995).

Hyperton-X, developed by Frank Mahony in 1982, primarily focuses on improving muscle functioning. It is applicable to chronic pain, accident trauma, stroke victims, athletic performance, learning problems, some emotional and other problems (Holdway, 1995).

Holographic repatterning (HR), an approach developed by Chloe Faith Wordsworth (1998), focuses on transforming unconscious patterns and beliefs. Through muscle checking, the therapist accesses the structure of the patient's unconscious patterns, and in this respect it is similar to many other kinesiological approaches. However, a multitude of treatment options are available, each of which is evaluated via muscle checking prior to its being administered to the patient. HR has similarities to TFH, One Brain, and a number of other approaches that Wordsworth studied. It is utilized to treat psychological and physical problems.

Specifically to address psychological concerns, psychotherapist and hypnotherapist Ann Howell developed *psyche-kinesiology* (PK) after studying kinesiology in the early 1970s (La Tourelle & Courtenay, 1992). Also in the 1970s, psychiatrist John Diamond developed a unique approach, *behavioral kinesiology* (BK), after studying with Goodheart, and clinical psychologist Roger Callahan developed his own approach, *Callahan Techniques–Thought Field Therapy*, after studying with Walther (1981, 1988), Blaich (1988), and Diamond. Other recent psychologically oriented approaches have included William F. Whisenant's *Psychological Kinesiology* (1990) and Robert M. Williams's Psych-K (*Free Yourself from Limiting Beliefs*, 1989). Also Tapas (Elizabeth) Fleming (1996), an acupuncturist with a background in kinesiology, has developed the *Tapas acupressure technique (TAT)*, which has been highly effective in the treatment of psychological trauma, allergies, and a number of other problems.

Of late, the history of kinesiology seems to be repeating itself, with a number of practitioners who studied with Callahan going off in their own directions. Among the roster are Patricia Carrington, Gary Craig, Judith Swack, and Larry Nims.

Carrington is the developer of *Acu-Tap* and the *releasing* method (1984, 1999). Acu-Tap is a simple, all-purpose treatment recipe or algorithm, based on some of Callahan's early work. She has found that this procedure yields a high success rate in alleviating psychological distress without having to specifically diagnose treatment points.

Craig's *emotional freedom techniques (EFT)* (Craig & Fowlie, 1995a, 1995b) entails one comprehensive therapeutic recipe or algorithm based on some of Callahan's later work, combined with questioning, "reminder phrases," and affirmations geared to access the significant aspects of the psychological problem. Additionally Craig offers what he calls the *palace of possibilities*, which involves the utilization of potent affirmations to facilitate personal achievement and the transmutation of limiting beliefs. Although Craig studied Callahan's diagnostic systems based on manual muscle testing and the *Voice Technology*[TM], his own method appears to successfully bypasses the need for precision diagnosis to a large extent.[2]

Swack (1994) has developed *healing from the body level up (HBLU)*, which entails detailed manual muscle testing in combination with methods from systematic applied kinesiology, neuro-linguistic programming, One Brain, and TFT. This method is reported to resolve trauma, emotional deprivation or injury, and physical problems.

Nims (1998) founded *Be Set Free Fast (BSFF)*, which entails a simple three-point algorithm combined with specific affirmations or pronouncements and basic manual muscle testing. He further installs positive beliefs by employing the temporal tap, a procedure explored by Goodheart. Nims has also developed what he calls instant BSFF, which attempts to program the patient's unconscious to go through the BSFF protocol whenever a problem develops.

Clinton (1999) has developed *matrix work*. Defining most dysfunction as having its origin in trauma, this energetic methodology focuses on the alleviation of trauma and repetitive traumatic patterns and the associated symptoms. Its reversal of negative core beliefs, desires, and fantasies is reported to transform basic character structure and thus treat personality disorders and many other conditions. This approach employs manual muscle testing to discern therapeutic needs. It addresses chakras as compared to acupoints to remove traumas and their sequelae and to promote the incorporation of positive core beliefs and positive qualities. Additionally meditation is employed to enhance and further the effects of energy work.

However, this is not intended to be a comprehensive listing of new directions in energetic psychotherapeutic approaches. There are also a variety of methods that work with chakras and other aspects of the human energy fields (Brennan, 1987, 1993; Hover-Kramer & Shames, 1997; Krieger, 1993; Laskow, 1992). The reader surely gets the idea that this area of treatment has been expanding exponentially. No doubt in time the politics of natural selection will determine which of the multitude of approaches survives and proliferates.

---

[2]See *Energy Psychology: Explorations at the Interface of Energy, Cognition, Behavior, and Health* (Gallo, 1998) for coverage on the Voice Technology[TM].

RESEARCH

The humble beginnings of a field involve impressions, the consensus of an increasingly visible group of professionals, and case studies. While these findings are gratifying, pique our interest, and serve to chart a course, they are insufficient for any field that hopes to develop scientifically. In time it is necessary to empirically evaluate the methodologies in more refined ways via single-case designs, randomized controlled trials, and eventually, systematic reviews of such trials. In these ways we come to a better understanding of what is operating within our methods. While we may believe deeply in the methods and techniques that we employ in the service of our patients, in the absence of closer scrutiny we cannot know with certainty what the active ingredients are.

However, it is also true that many of the methods described herein are not easily evaluated with traditional research designs. In many instances the variables studied in behavioral science designs are quite limited and easily subjected to the test, although the richness of the individual's experience is no doubt neglected in the process. While it may be easy enough to evaluate the effectiveness of the negative affect erasing method (NAEM), the healing energy light process (HELP), or algorithms described elsewhere (Gallo, 1998) in the treatment of trauma, phobias, clinical depression and so forth, the therapeutic effects achieved via energy diagnostics is an entirely different matter. In the latter instance, variability among therapists, protocols, derived energy configurations associated with various problems, therapist-patient match, and so on results in considerable complexity. Therefore, phenomenological research methods and single-case designs are useful adjuncts to the overall research approach, incorporating the human experience into our designs (Giorgi, 1970) and offering noteworthy insights.

Some may argue the age-old position that an approach should not be employed until the efficacy studies have supported and defined the limits of the approach. And yet if we survey the health art-sciences, it is apparent that this can never be the case. Many approaches develop out in the field and are later scrutinized and hopefully refined in the laboratory. Moreover, the human condition is such that suffering demands our compassionate attention. When we, as clinicians, realize that an approach increases our effectiveness in helping patients, are we to set it on the shelf and await the efficacy studies? I think not. This is not intended to be a disparaging refrain about research, but rather a recognition of the human problems to which we must offer effective and efficient solutions on a daily basis.

ETHICAL CONSIDERATIONS

A number of unique ethical considerations arise as a result of this methodology. An obvious concern is the issue of physical touch. While the therapist's physical contact with the patient is quite limited when conducting the diagnostic procedures described in this text, some contact is needed to obtain an accurate diagnosis. While the contact is generally limited to touching a patient's wrist, hand, or shoulder in order to evaluate muscle firmness, a degree of caution is warranted. Obviously, the patient's permission is needed for both etiquette and ethical reasons.

As an aside, it should be noted that many therapeutic approaches entail some degree of acceptable touch. For example, some approaches to hypnotic induction involve touch, and surely the biofeedback therapist touches the patient to some degree. In addition, when a patient is experiencing inordinate distress, is it not proper and humanistic to authentically offer a caring touch on a hand or a shoulder? Touch is not invariably improper.

However, since at the present time there are jurisdictional restrictions on the therapist regarding any degree of touch, it is recommended that the therapist focus on developing intuitive diagnostic skills. For example, the protocols in Chapter 7 can be conducted without needing to have physical contact with the patient. If the therapist correctly intuits that the disruption is related primarily to a specific meridian, having the patient stimulate that meridian at a variety of points will often achieve significant results.[3] Psychological reversal and neurologic disorganization can also often be assumed on the basis of clinical observation, and the patient can then be directed through the correction phases.

It is incumbent upon the therapist-examiner to pursue adequate training in these methods before pursuing them with patients. While texts of this nature are useful adjuncts, they are no substitute for comprehensive training. Obviously, this is a specialty area.

One additional ethical consideration is the issue of informed consent. It is the therapist's responsibility to make the patient aware that while these methods have been found to be highly effective and efficient clinically, the currently available empirical research is rather limited. Further, it is recommended that the therapist incorporate these methods into a compre-

---

[3] Some therapists have found that surrogate testing, themselves being the surrogate, has yielded effective therapeutic results. This approach also warrants empirical research.

hensive treatment plan that includes other psychotherapeutic components. The protocols discussed herein are always nested within a framework that includes respect for and acceptance of the client, thought recognition, externalization of the problem, patient assignments, and other ingredients contained in effective psychotherapeutic approaches in general.

THE FUTURE OF ENERGY PSYCHOLOGY

Energy psychology is a rapidly evolving discipline. In this and my previous work (Gallo, 1998) I have specified a number of techniques and protocols that have been found to be effective in treating a wide range of psychological problems and even peak performance issues. In their development, every effort has been made to ensure methodological consistency. In addition to clinically exploring the benefits of this approach, it is now the time to conduct detailed empirical investigations. Documentation is needed in order to assist our profession in harnessing the benefits that these methods have to offer.

GLOSSARY

acupoint Acupuncture point. Points on the surface of the skin, many of which evidence lower electrical resistance relative to adjacent skin surface. It is thought that subtle energy from the environment enters the body through these portals. The acupoints interconnect along meridians.

alarm points Meridian diagnostic points located bilaterally and along the midline of the torso. Also referred to as test points.

amygdala An almond-shaped brain structure within the limbic system, instrumental in emotional expression.

applied kinesiology (AK) A system using muscle testing as functional neurology, concerned primarily with neuromuscular function as it relates to the structural, chemical, and mental physiologic regulatory mechanisms. AK has multidisciplinary applications.

attunement Tuning in or accessing a thought field.

aura The energetic field that surrounds and permeates the body. Also referred to as biofield. It is hypothesized that the aura is composed of several distinct layers.

biofield *See* aura.

chakra Body energy centers that serve as transformers of subtle energies. The chakras are assumed to convert subtle energy into chemical and cellular forms. Chakra is from the Sanskrit, meaning "wheel."

cranial faults Failure of the skull bones to move in its normal, rhythmic manner.

cross-crawl exercises Originally developed by Doman and Delacato (Delacato, 1966), and elaborated further in applied kinesiology and various AK offshoots such as educational kinesiology, these exercises are often useful in the treatment of neurologic disorganization, learning disabilities, and as an adjunct to various energy psychology procedures.

215

energy psychology The branch of psychology that studies the effects of energy systems, such as the acupuncture meridians and morphic resonance, on emotions and behavior.

energy psychotherapy Psychotherapeutic approaches that specifically address bioenergy systems in the diagnosis and treatment of psychological problems.

energy toxin Substances that deleteriously affect the bioenergy system. When an energy toxin is significantly affecting the patient's energy system, therapeutic results can be blocked.

hemisphere dominance test (HDT) A therapy localization procedure that assists the examiner in discerning relative cerebral hemispheric dominance and localizing affected meridians.

in the clear Testing a muscle without concurrent therapy localization or introducing factors that can otherwise influence the muscle to respond as either weak or strong.

indicator muscle A muscle that is isolated to gauge change in strength or in response to a stimulus.

meridian A channel or pathway that carries subtle energy through the body, interconnected with acupoints. There are 12 primary meridians, 2 collector meridians, and 6 additional extraordinary channels.

muscular units of distress (MUD) Similar to subjective units of distress (SUD), MUD is a measure of an indicator muscle's response to an inquiry of the subject's level of distress in a particular context. A comparison of the SUD and MUD measures provides additional information that is not available from either alone.

neurologic disorganization A condition that involves the central nervous system's misinterpreting and misconstruing nerve impulses. When this condition is present, the effectiveness of manual muscle testing is impaired. Also referred to as switching.

neurolymphatic reflex Originally identified by Chapman (Walther, 1988), these reflexes are primarily located between the ribs and in the pelvic region. Stimulation of the reflexes promote lymphatic drainage.

neurovascular reflex Originally identified by Bennett (Walther, 1988), stimulation of these reflexes actuate circulation in various locations throughout the body.

ocular lock A useful screening indicator of neurologic disorganization, characterized by the failure of the eyes to work together and often evidenced by a saccadic movement of the eyes at some point along a 360° rotation.

perturbation Proposed fundamental subtle energetic catalysts of negative emotions. Perturbations are correlated with specific acupoints.

psychological reversal "A state or condition that prevents healing and blocks otherwise effective treatments from working, [u]sually accompanied by negative attitudes and self-sabotage that leads to self-defeating behavior" (Callahan & Perry, 1991, p. 221).

pulse testing   A method of testing the hypersensitivity of an individual to an exogenous substance.

resonance   In physics, the increase in amplitude of oscillation of a system (electrical or mechanical) exposed to a force whose frequency approximates or equals the frequency of the system. In energy therapies, this phenomenon relates to the energetic field associated with thought fields and emotions.

resonance lock   To attune and entrain or lock-in a thought field. This is often accomplished by imagining or otherwise thinking about an emotionally charged issue, although sustained resonance can be achieved via various procedures such as the leg lock or glabella tap.

strong muscle   During muscle testing, the muscle functions neurologically to its capacity and immediately locks.

subjective units of distress (SUD)   A term coined by Joseph Wolpe indicating a subject-report measure of distress level on a scale such as 0 to 10 or 1 to 10.

switching   *See* neurologic disorganization.

temporal sphenoidal (TS) line   "Described by the border of the temporal and sphenoidal bones, the temporal border of the zygomatic bones, and the superior border of the zygomatic arch. Palpable nodules along this line are indicative of corresponding muscular weaknesses" (Walther, 1988, p. 558).

temporal tap   A method for interrupting the brain's sensory filtering so as to assess therapeutic effectiveness, to improve muscle responsiveness, to modify habitual patterns, or to install beliefs.

therapy localization   A diagnostic procedure whereby the subject is directed to place his/her hand or fingers at a specific location on the body while an indicator muscle is tested to determine changes in muscle responsiveness. Therapy localization is an aspect of the diagnostic process and must be combined with additional clinical and empirical tests in order to arrive at a valid conclusion.

thought field   While thought entails sensory, linguistic, neurologic, and chemical features, thought field indicates that thought also entails an energetic field, probably electromagnetic to a large extent.

triad of health   Structural, chemical, and mental/emotional factors that can result in health consequences when not in balance. The health triad is an essential consideration in holistic approaches.

weak muscle   During muscle testing, the muscle does not function neurologically to its capacity. This is a measure of muscle responsiveness, not muscle integrity.

BIBLIOGRAPHY

Alexander, F., & French, T. (1946). *Psychoanalytic theory*. New York: Ronald Press.

American Psychiatric Association. (1994). *Diagnostic and statistical manual of mental disorders* (4th ed.). Washington, DC: Author.

Andreas, C., & Andreas, S. (1995). *Eye movement integration (applied with a Vietnam Veteran who has been experiencing intrusive memories)* [Videotape]. Boulder, CO: NLP Comprehensive.

Bandler, R., & Grinder, J. (1975). *Patterns of the hypnotic techniques of Milton H. Erickson, M.D.* (Vol. I). Cupertino, CA: Meta.

Bandler, R., & Grinder, J. (1979). *Frogs into princes: Neuro-linguistic programming*. Moab, UT: Real People.

Beardall, A. G. (1982). *Clinical kinesiology instruction manual*. Lake Oswego, OR: Author.

Beardall, A. G. (1995). *Clinical kinesiology laboratory manual*. Portland, OR: Human Bio-Dynamics.

Becker, R. O. (1990). *Cross currents*. New York: Putnam.

Becker, R. O., Reichmanis, M., & Marino, A. (1976). Electrophysiological correlates of acupuncture points and meridians. *Psychoenergetic Systems, 1*(105), 195–212.

Becker, R. O., & Selden, G. (1985). *The body electric*. New York: Morrow.

Beyens, F. (1998). Reinterpretation of traditional concepts in acupuncture. In J. Filshie & A. White (Eds.), *Medical acupuncture: A Western scientific approach* (pp. 391–407). Edinburgh: Churchill Livingstone.

Bingham, W., & Moore, B. (1959). *How to interview*. New York: Harper & Row.

Blaich, R. M. (1988, Winter). Applied kinesiology and human performance. *Collected Papers of International College of Applied Kinesiology*
(pp. 7–15). Shawnee Mission, KS: International College of Applied Kinesiology.

Bohm, D. (1980). *Wholeness and the implicate order.* Boston: Routledge &
Kegan Paul.

Brennan, B. A. (1987). *Hands of light.* New York: Bantam.

Brennan, B. A. (1993). *Light emerging.* New York: Bantam.

Burr, H. S. (1972). *Blueprint for immortality: The electric patterns of life.*
Essex, England: Saffron Walden.

Callahan, R. J. (1981, Winter). Psychological reversal. *Collected Papers
of the International College of Applied Kinesiology* (pp. 79–96). Shawnee
Mission, KS: International College of Applied Kinesiology.

Callahan, R. J. (1985). *Five minute phobia cure.* Wilmington, DE: Enter-
prise.

Callahan, R. J. (1990). *The rapid treatment of panic, agoraphobia, and
anxiety.* Indian Wells, CA: Author.

Callahan, R. J., & Callahan, J. (1996). *Thought field therapy and trauma:
Treatment and theory.* Indian Wells, CA: Author.

Callahan, R. J., & Perry, P. (1991). *Why do I eat when I'm not hungry?*
New York: Doubleday.

Carlson, R., & Bailey, J. (1997). *Slowing down to the speed of life.* New
York: HarperCollins.

Carrington, P. (1984). *Releasing.* New York: Morrow.

Carrington, P. (1999). *The power of letting go.* Boston: Elements.

Charny, J. E. (1966). Psychosomatic manifestations of rapport in psychotherapy. *Psychosomatic Medicine, 28*(4), 305–315.

Chen, E. (1995). *Cross-sectional anatomy of acupoints.* Hong Kong:
Longman.

Clinton, N. A. (1999). *Matrix work manual.* Princeton, NJ: Author.

Condon, W. S. (1970). Methods of microanalysis of sound films of behavior. *Behavior Research Methods and Instruments, 2*(2), 51–54.

Cooper, N. A., & Clum, G. A. (1989). Imaginal flooding as a supplemen-
tary treatment for PTSD in combat veterans: a controlled study. *Behavior
Therapy, 20*, 381–391.

Cordaro, L., & Ison, J. R. (1963). Psychology of the scientist: X. Observer
bias in classical conditioning of the planarian. *Psychological Reports, 13*,
787–789.

Craig, G., & Fowlie, A. (1995a). *Emotional freedom techniques: The manual.* Sea Ranch, CA: Author.

Craig, G., & Fowlie, A. (1995b). *Emotional freedom techniques: The complete course.* Sea Ranch, CA: Author.

Cutler, E. W. (1997). *Winning the war against asthma and allergies.* New York: Delmar.

Delacato, C. H. (1966). *The diagnosis and treatment of speech and reading problems.* Springfield, IL: Charles C. Thomas.

Dennison, P. (1981). *Switching on.* Glendale, CA: Edu-Kinesthetics.

Dennison, P., & Dennison, G. (1987). *Edu-K for kids.* Glendale, CA: Edu-Kinesthetics.

Dennison, P. E., & Dennison, G. (1989). *Brain gym handbook.* Ventura, CA: Educational Kinesiology Foundation.

Diamond, J. (1978). *Behavioral kinesiology and the autonomic nervous system.* New York: Institute of Behavioral Kinesiology.

Diamond, J. (1979). *Behavioral kinesiology.* New York: Harper & Row.

Diamond, J. (1980a). *The collected papers of John Diamond, M.D.* (Vol. II). New York: Archaeus.

Diamond, J. (1980b). *Your body doesn't lie.* New York: Warner.

Diamond, J. (1985). *Life energy.* New York: Dodd, Mead.

Diamond, J. (1988). *Life-energy analysis: A way to cantillation.* Valley Cottage, NY: Archaeus.

Dickes, R. (1975). Technical considerations of the therapeutic and working alliances. *International Journal of Psychoanalytic Psychotherapy, 4,* 1–24.

Diepold, J. (1998). *Touch and breathe: An alternative treatment approach with meridian based psychotherapies.* New Jersey: Author.

Dilts, R. B., Grinder, J., Bandler, R., DeLozier, J., & Cameron-Bandler, L. (1979). *Neuro-linguistic programming, I.* Cupertino, CA: Meta.

Dossey, L. (1989). *Recovering the soul: A scientific and spiritual search.* New York: Bantam.

Dossey, L. (1993). *Healing words: The power of prayer and the practice of medicine.* San Francisco: HarperCollins.

Durlacher, J. V. (1994). *Freedom from fear forever.* Tempe, AZ: Van Ness.

Epston, D., & White, M. (1992). *Experience, contradiction, narrative and imagination.* Alelaide, Australia: Dulwich Centre.

Erikson, E. H. (1959). Identity and the life cycle. *Psychological Issues, 1*(1). (Published in paperback by Norton, 1980).

Fiedler, F. (1950). The concept of an ideal therapeutic relationship. *Journal of Consulting Psychology, 14,* 239–245.

Filshie, J., & White, A. (1998). *Medical acupuncture: A Western scientific approach.* Edinburgh: Churchill Livingstone.

Fleming, T. (1996). *Reduce traumatic stress in minutes: The Tapas acupressure technique (TAT) workbook.* Torrance, CA: Tapas Fleming.

Freud, S. (1958). *The standard edition of the complete psychological works of Sigmund Freud.* New York: Norton.

Furman, M., & Gallo, F. (2000). *The neurophysics of human behavior: Explorations at the interface of the brain, mind, behavior, and information.* Boca Raton: CRC.

Gallo, F. (1994a). *Thought field therapy level 1 (and associated methods): Training manual.* Hermitage, PA: Author.

Gallo, F. (1994b). *Thought field therapy level 2 (and associated methods): Training manual.* Hermitage, PA: Author.

Gallo, F. (1996a). Reflections on active ingredients in efficient treatments of PTSD, Part 1. *Electronic Journal of Traumatology,* 2(1). Available: http://www.fsu.edu/~trauma/>

Gallo, F. (1996b). Reflections on active ingredients in efficient treatments of PTSD, Part 2. *Electronic Journal of Traumatology,* 2(2). Available: http://www.fsu.edu/~trauma/>

Gallo, F. (1996c, June). Therapy by energy. *Anchor Point,* 46–51.

Gallo, F. (1997a). A no-talk cure for trauma: Thought field therapy violates all the rules. *Family Therapy Networker,* 21(2), 65–75.

Gallo, F. (1997b). *Energy diagnostic and treatment methods (EDxTM): Basic training manual.* Hermitage, PA: Author.

Gallo, F. (1998). *Energy psychology: Explorations at the interface of energy, cognition, behavior, and health.* Boca Raton: CRC.

Gallo, F. (1999). A no-talk cure for trauma: Thought field therapy violates all the rules. In R. Simon, L. Markowitz, C. Barrilleaux, & B. Topping (Eds.), *The art of psychotherapy: Case studies from the family therapy networker* (pp. 244–255). New York: John Wiley & Sons.

Garten, H. (1996, December). The mechanism of muscle test reactions and challenge in applied kinesiology: An attempt to explain the test phenomena. (Revised by F. Annunciato, Neurobiology Laboratory, Dept. Of Histology, University of Sao Paulo, Brazil). *Townsend Letter for Doctors and Patients.*

Gazzaniga, M. (1967). The split brain in man. *Scientific American,* 217, 24–29.

Gazzaniga, M. (1985). *The social brain.* New York: Basic.

Gerber, R. (1988). *Vibrational medicine.* Santa Fe, NM: Bear.

Giorgi, A. (1970). *Psychology as a human science: A phenomenologically based approach.* New York: Harper & Row.

Goldstein, A. P., & Shipman, W. G. (1961). Patient expectancies, symptom reduction and aspects of the initial psychotherapeutic interview. *Journal of Clinical Psychology, 17,* 129–133.

Goodheart, G. J. (1987). *You'll be better.* Geneva, OH: Author.

Goswami, A. (1993). *The self-aware universe: How consciousness creates the material world.* New York: Tarcher.

Gunn, C. C. (1998). Acupuncture in context. In J. Filshie & A. White (Eds.), *Medical acupuncture: A Western scientific approach* (pp. 11–16). Edinburgh: Churchill Livingstone.

Hallbom, T., & Smith, S. (1988). *Eliminating allergies* [videotape]. Boulder, CO: NLP Comprehensive.

Holdway, A. (1995). *Kinesiology: Muscle testing & energy balancing for health & well-being.* Rockport, MA: Element.

Hover-Kramer, D., & Shames, K. H. (1997). *Energetic approaches to emotional healing.* New York: Delmar.

Hunt, V. (1989). *Infinite mind: Science of the human vibrations of consciousness.* Malibu, CA: Malibu.

Jaffe, J. (1967). Verbal behavior analysis in psychiatric interviews with the aid of digital computers. *Disorders of Communication: Association for Research in Nervous and Mental Disease, 42,* 389–399.

Johnson, R. (1994). *Rapid eye technology.* Salem, OR: RainTree.

Keane, T. M., Fairbank, J. A., Caddell, J. M., & Zimmering, R. T. (1989). Implosive (flooding) therapy reduces symptoms of PTSD in Vietnam combat veterans. *Behavior Therapy, 20,* 245–260.

Kendall, H. O., & Kendall, F. M. P. (1949). *Muscles: Testing and function.* Baltimore: Williams & Wilkins.

Kendall, H., Kendall, F., & Wadsworth, G. (1971). *Muscle testing and function* (2nd ed.). Baltimore: Williams & Wilkins.

Kendall, F. M. P., & McCreary, E. K. (1993). *Muscles: Testing and function.* Baltimore: Williams & Wilkins.

Kendon, A. (1970a). Some relationships between body motion and speech. In A. W. Siegman & B. Pope (Eds.), *Studies in dyadic communication* (pp. 177–210). New York: Pergamon.

Kendon, A. (1970b). Movement coordination in social interaction. *Acta Psychologica, 32,* 100–125.

Koestler, A. (1967). *The ghost in the machine.* London: Hutchinson & Co.

Krieger, D. (1993). *Accepting your power to heal.* Santa Fe, NM: Bear.

Kuhn, T. S. (1962). *The structure of scientific revolutions.* Chicago: University of Chicago.

La Tourelle, M., & Courtenay, A. (1992). *Thorsons introductory guide to kinesiology.* London: Thorsons.

Langman, L. (1972). The implications of the electro-metric test in cancer of the female genital tract. In H. S. Burr (Ed.), *Blueprint for immortality: The electric patterns of life* (pp. 137–154). Essex, England: Saffron Walden.

Laskow, L. (1992). *Healing with love.* San Francisco: HarperCollins.

Lawson, A., & Calderon, L. (1997). Interexaminer reliability of applied kinesiology manual muscle testing. *Perceptual Motor Skills, 84,* 539–546.

Leisman, G., Shambaugh, P., & Ferentz, A. (1989). Somatosensory evoked potential changes during muscle testing. *International Journal of Neuroscience, 45,* 143–151.

Lennard, H. L., & Bernstein, A. (1960). *The anatomy of psychotherapy.* New York: Columbia University.

Levy, S. L., & Lehr, C. (1996). *Your body can talk.* Prescott, AZ: Hohm.

MacKinnon, R. A., & Michels, R. (1971). *The psychiatric interview in clinical practice.* Philadelphia: Saunders.

Matarazzo, J. D., Weitman, M., Saslow, G., & Wiens, A. N. (1963). Interviewer influence on duration of interviewee speech. *Journal of Verbal Learning and Verbal Behavior, 1,* 451–458.

Menninger, K. (1958). *Theory of psychoanalytic technique.* New York: Basic.

Mills, R. (1995). *Health realization.* New York: Sulburger & Graham.

Nambudripad, D. S. (1993). *Say goodbye to illness.* Buena Park, CA: Delta.

Natale, M. (1975). Convergence of mean vocal intensity in dyadic communication as a function of social desirability. *Journal of Personality and Social Psychology, 32*(5), 790–804.

Nathanson, D. L. (1992). *Shame and pride: Affect, sex, and the birth of the self.* New York: Norton.

Nims, L. P. (1998). *Be set free fast: Training manual.* Orange, CA: Author.

Nordenstrom, B. (1983). *Biologically closed electric circuits: Clinical, experimental, and theoretical evidence for an additional circulatory system.* Stockholm: Nordic.

O'Hanlon, B., & Wilk, J. (1987). *Shifting contexts: The generation of effective psychotherapy.* New York: Guilford.

Palmer, D. D. (1910). *The science, art, and philosophy of chiropractic.* Portland, OR: Portland.

Pitman, R. K., Altman, B., Greenwald, E., Longpre, R. E., Macklin, M. L., Poire, R. E., & Steketee, G. S. (1991). Psychiatric complications during flooding therapy for posttraumatic stress disorder. *Journal of Clinical Psychiatry, 52,* 17–20.

Pomeranz, B. (1996). Acupuncture and the raison d'etre for alternative medicine. *Alternative Therapies, 2*(6), 84–91.

Pransky, G. S. (1992). *The relationship handbook.* Blue Ridge Summit, PA: HIS & TAB.

Pransky, G. S. (1998). *The renaissance of psychology.* New York: Sultzburger & Graham.

Rapp, D. (1986). *The impossible child.* Buffalo, NY: Practical Allergy Research Foundation.

Rapp, D. (1991). *Is this your child? Discovering and treating unrecognized allergies in children and adults.* New York: Morrow.

Reichmanis, M., Andrew, A., & Becker, R. O. (1975). Electrical correlates of acupuncture points. *IEEE Trans Biomedical Engineering, 22,* 203–216.

Reichmanis, M., Andrew, A., & Becker, R. O. (1976). DC skin conductance variation at acupuncture loci. *American Journal of Chinese Medicine, 4,* 69–72.

Rochlitz, S. (1995). *Allergies and candida.* Mahopac, NY: Human Ecology Balancing Sciences.

Rogers, C. (1942a). *Counseling and psychotherapy.* Boston: Houghton Mifflin.

Rogers, C. (1942b). *Client-centered therapy.* Boston: Houghton Mifflin.

Rogers, C. (1957). The necessary and sufficient conditions of therapeutic personality change. *Journal of Consulting Psychology, 21*(2), 95–103.

Rosenthal, R., & Fode, K. L. (1963). The effects of experimenter bias on the performance of albino rats. *Psychological Reports, 12,* 491–511.

Rosenthal, R., & Jacobson, L. (1966). Teachers' expectancies; determinants of pupils' IQ gains. *Psychological Reports, 19,* 115–118.

Rosenthal, R., & Lawson, R. (1964). A longitudinal study of the effects of experimenter bias on the operant learning of laboratory rats. *Journal of Psychiatric Research, 2,* 61–72.

Scheflen, A. E. (1964a). Communication and regulation in psychotherapy. *Psychiatry, 27*(4), 126–136.

Scheflen, A. E. (1964b). The significance of posture in communication systems. *Psychiatry, 27*(4), 316–331.

Scheflen, A. E. (1965). Quasi-courtship behavior in psychotherapy. *Psychiatry, 28,* 245–257.

Schiffer, F. (1998). *Of two minds: The revolutionary science of dual brain psychology*. New York: Free.

Schofield, W. (1964). *Psychotherapy: The purchase of friendship*. Englewood Cliffs, NJ: Prentice-Hall.

Scott, J. (1988). *Cure your own allergies in minutes*. San Francisco, CA: Health Kinesiology.

Shapiro, F. (1995). *Eye movement desensitization and reprocessing: Basic principles, protocols, and procedures*. New York: Guilford.

Sheldrake, R. (1981). *A new science of life*. Los Angeles: Tarcher.

Sheldrake, R. (1988). *The presence of the past*. New York: Times.

Shobin, M. Z. (1980). *An investigation of the effect of verbal pacing on initial therapeutic rapport*. Ann Arbor, MI: University Microfilms International.

Stokes, G., & Whiteside, D. (1981). *Touch for health midday — Midnight law and the five elements rebalancing*. Pasadena, CA: T. H. Enterprises.

Stux, G., & Pomeranz, B. (1995). *Basics of acupuncture* (3rd ed.). New York: Springer.

Sullivan, H. S. (1954). *The psychiatric interview*. New York: Norton.

Swack, J. (1994, March). The basic structure of loss and violence trauma imprints. *Anchor Point.*

Talbot, M. (1991). *The holographic universe*. New York: HarperCollins.

Teeguarden, I. M. (1996). *A complete guide to acupressure*. Tokyo: Japan Publications.

Thie, J. F. (1973). *Touch for health*. Pasadena, CA: T.H. Enterprises.

Thomas, C. L. (1973). *Taber's cyclopedic medical dictionary*. Philadelphia: F. A. Davis.

Tiller, W. A. (1997). *Science and human transformation: Subtle energies, intentionality and consciousness*. California: Pavior.

Travis, C. B., McLean, B. E., & Ribar, C. (Eds). (1989). Environmental toxins: Psychological, behavioral, and sociocultural aspects, 1973–1989. *PsycINFO*, 5. Washington, DC: American Psychological Association.

Truax, C. B. (1961). A scale for the measurement of accurate empathy. *Psychiatric Institute Bulletin, 1*, 12.

Truax, C. B. (1963). Effective ingredients in psychotherapy: an approach to unravelling the patient-therapist interaction. *Journal of Counseling Psychology, 10*(3), 256–263

van Gigch, J. P. (1974). *Applied general systems theory*. New York: Harper & Row.

de Vernejoul, P., Albarède, P., & Darras, J. C. (1985). Etude des meridiens d'acupuncture par les traceurs radioactifs [Study of the acupuncture meridians with radioactive tracers]. *Bulletin of the Academy of National Medicine (Paris), 169,* 1071–1075.

Wallace, L. (1974). The psychoanalytic situation and the transference neurosis. *Israel Annals of Psychiatry and Related Disciplines, 12*(4), 304–318.

Walther, D. S. (1981). *Applied kinesiology: Vol. I. Basic procedures and muscle testing.* Pueblo, CO: Systems DC.

Walther, D. S. (1988). *Applied kinesiology: Synopsis.* Pueblo, CO: Systems DC.

Webb, J. T. (1970). Interview synchrony: An investigation of two speech rate measures in an automated standard interview. In A. W. Siegman & B. Pope (Eds.), *Studies in dyadic communication* (pp. 115–133). New York: Pergamon.

Whisenant, W. F. (1990). *Psychological kinesiology: Changing the body's beliefs.* Austin, TX: Monarch Butterfly Productions.

Wiens, A. N., Saslow, G., & Matarazzo, J. D. (1966). Speech interruption behavior during interviews. *Psychotherapy: Theory, Research and Practice, 3,* 153–156.

Williams, R. (1989). *Free yourself from limiting beliefs* [videotape]. Denver, CO: American Magnetic Media.

Wordsworth, C. (1998). *Scientific principles of holographic repatterning.* Albuquerque, NM: Author.

Yang, Jwing-Ming. (1989). *The roots of Chinese qigong.* Jamaica Plain, MA: YMAA.

Young, A. (1976a). *The reflexive universe: Evolution of consciousness.* Lake Oswego, OR: Robert Briggs.

Young, A. (1976b). *The geometry of meaning.* Mill Valley, CA: Robert Briggs.

Young, A. (1984). *The foundations of science: The missing parameter.* San Francisco: Robert Briggs.

Zetzel, E. (1956). Current concepts of transference. *International Journal of Psychoanalysis, 37,* 369–376.

Zmiewski, P., Wiseman, N., & Ellis, A. (1985). *Fundamentals of Chinese medicine.* Brookline, MA: Paradigm.

Zukav, G. (1979). *The dancing wu li masters: An overview of the new physics.* New York: Bantam.

INDEX